'Andy McCann gives a unique, and highly informative account from his own life experience of a stroke, together with his inspirational story of the challenging journey through recovery. Andy also presents current biological information about strokes in an easily assimilated format, which is augmented by additional stories from stroke survivors. This book is not only a highly valuable source of information for anyone who has suffered a stroke, but also those wishing to understand the contributing factors and possible consequences. Andy's book also offers many approaches to establishing a healthier and more balanced life style. A thoroughly well worth read.'

– Gavin Emerson, Director of Academic Studies,
Brief Strategic Therapy and Clinical Hypnosis (BST) Foundation

'In this book Andy has managed to include so much information crucial to people who have survived a stroke and their families and yet has kept a personal touch which makes the book both readable and enjoyable. A must-read for anyone whose life has been affected by stroke. Inspirational and informative."

– Dr Tig Calvert, Senior Lecturer in Neuropsychologyand Clinical Hypnotherapist,
St Mary's College, University of Surrey

'A very personal and motivating account of a stroke recovery with lots of useful information and insight for people who have had a stroke and their families and friends.'

– Dr Cliff Arnall, Psychologist, Cardiff University

'This book has helped me on three levels: first, as a medically interested person, the frank and clear way in which the stroke event is described, with the medical terms explained, has indeed made me realise we all have a gap in our knowledge to fill about this issue; second, as a therapist, it has given me a unique insight into the stroke survivor that has enabled me now to fully appreciate the emotional and physical trauma suffered, allowing me to adjust my massage treatment accordingly in the future for the better; and lastly, as a friend of Andy's for nearly 20 years, the book gives me the missing pieces I didn't know were missing, of why he is my friend. An inspirational "textbook for the unaware" explaining the lessons to be learned for all of us that "live life in the fast lane" and who "expect it to happen to someone else". Life is not a rehearsal and we must all take the necessary proactive steps to ensure we keep our good health.'

– Paul Harris, Sports Massage Therapist

'Highly informative text, which will be a valuable educational resource. Raising the profile of stroke as a "brain attack" and enhancing the need for us all to follow a personal stroke prevention programme. The use of medical terminology has been integrated enabling understanding across the range of medical expertise. Rehabilitation procedures are thought-provoking, inspirational and an excellent example of positive thinking.'

— *Neil Perkins, Head of Physical Education, Cardinal Newman School*

'This book provides an alternative viewpoint on stroke survival. Although there are many medical references and textbooks outlining the underlying medical conditions associated with stroke, this book provides valuable information, which is complementary to the available medical literature. The author, as a result of his own experiences, has compiled an informative text on many issues related to our understanding of stroke and the effect it has on life "post-event".

… This book provides readers with a "positive attitude" approach to the problems experienced by stroke survivors of all ages and gender, highlights alternative information previously not available for stroke victims and outlines the benefits of traditional and alternative exercise, eating healthy food and suggests that stroke survivors can move on to lead full, complete and rewarding lives.

… The author has…written a definitive text, which includes material that can be utilised to improve and enhance the mental and physical quality of life experienced by stroke victims. Stroke prevention has become his passion so others can become proactive, rather than reactive. The author knows that he has, forever, been changed by his "stroke of misfortune" but has emerged producing a "stroke of genius".'

— *Dr Julien Steven Baker, Reader in Applied Physiology, Health and Exercise Science Research Unit, University of Glamorgan*

'I am delighted to be able to introduce a book which not only speaks of the experiences of the author, but includes contributions from many other stroke survivors describing what has helped – and hindered – their recovery.

Stroke affects more than 10,000 people under the age of 55 every year in the UK, but young stroke survivors are still often bundled into geriatric wards and given little help. Andy shows just what can be achieved through determination and grit!'

— *Christina Meacham, Chief Executive, Different Strokes*

Stroke Survivor

A Personal Guide to Coping and Recovery

Andy McCann

Forewords by Robin Sieger and The Stroke Association (UK)

Jessica Kingsley Publishers
London and Philadelphia

First published in 2006
by Jessica Kingsley Publishers
116 Pentonville Road
London N1 9JB, UK
and
400 Market Street, Suite 400
Philadelphia, PA 19106, USA

www.jkp.com

Library of Congress Cataloging in Publication Data

McCann, Andy, 1966-
    Stroke survivor : a personal guide to recovery / Andy McCann ; foreword by Robin Sieger ; foreword by the Stroke Association.-- 1st American pbk. ed.
        p. cm.
    Includes bibliographical references and index.
    ISBN-13: 978-1-84310-410-0 (pbk. : alk. paper)
        ISBN-10: 1-84310-410-5 (pbk. : alk. paper)   1. McCann, Andy 1966---Health. 2. Cerebrovascular disease--Patients--Biography. 3. Cerebrovascular disease--Patients--Rehabilitation. I. Title.

    RC388.5.M25 2006
    362.196'810092--dc22

                                                                            2005029510

British Library Cataloguing in Publication Data
A CIP catalogue record for this book is available from the British Library

ISBN-13: 978 1 84310 410 0
ISBN-10: 1 84310 410 5

Printed and bound in Great Britain by
Athenaeum Press, Gateshead, Tyne and Wear

To Mum and Dad

Sorry you have had to support me
through so much
…and for so long!

To Anne

'To the world you might be one person,
but to one person you might be the world.'

(Anon.)

Contents

List of Figures

List of Tables

Acknowledgements

My first acknowledgement must go to Anne. The details of her support are described in the text, but perhaps even this is not an adequate way of thanking her for her support. Thanks go to my closest friends, both near and far, and I know that no more need be said. However, I am grateful to Mark and Paul for being so physically close at my time of need (and to Mark for being on hand again, to help me with the IT needed to write this book). Thanks also to my former colleagues at Cardinal Newman School for helping me believe that I still have a lot to offer, and especially Kate who also supported me with the 'administrative transition' out of teaching.

I must thank my GP, Dr Guy Marshal, for the continuous support and understanding, but most of all for making me feel like I was his only patient. Thanks also to my consultants, Dr Shetty and Dr Ghosh, for the reassurances. In addition, special thanks must go to my therapists for the physical therapy and stimulating dialogue. These are Steve Cannon, Chartered Physiotherapist of the Diagnostic Treatment and Rehabilitation (DTR) Clinic in Cardiff; Paul Harris of One-to-One Sports Therapy in Cardiff (also for his contribution to the section on sports massage therapy in Chapter 10); and Judith Whately, Principal Reflexologist at Something Else in Merthyr Tydfil. Equally importantly, thanks to everyone whose varied expressions of support were timely enough to help me look to the future. These include Terri Williams, from the Cardiff Regional Office (the Stroke Association); Andrew Dickenson (the charity Different Strokes); Robin Sieger (Sieger International, especially for that first personal email and gift); Alun James (for the looking after the jobs around the house); Gareth Rees (RCT School Improvement Division); and Paul Fielding (Cambria Financial).

I would like to thank Rick Moneymaker and Tom Muncy of Dragon Society International (DSI) for allowing me to use the phrase 'players to the game' in the context of this book. Thanks also to the Brief & Strategic Therapy Foundation for providing a stimulating and practical course and high level of training in clinical and medical hypnotherapy. The skills will stay with me for life.

I would also like to thank and acknowledge Maggie Alexander, Chief Executive of the Brain and Spine Association (www.brainandspine.org.uk), for her personal co-operation; the Brain and Spine Foundation and Philip Wilson FMAA RMIP for permission to reproduce Figures 7.1, 7.6 and 8.1; Victoria Gill, Administrator for the British Neuroscience Association (www.bna.org.uk), for her personal co-operation; and Professor Richard Morris for allowing the reproduction of Figure 7.4. Every effort has been made to obtain permission for copyright material and, as far as is possible, all other sources of contribution are acknowledged in the references. Of course, in all cases errors and interpretation are my responsibility alone.

A special thank you to Jessica Kingsley Publishers for publishing this work, and to Stephen Jones of JKP for his support and advice throughout the months. I would also like to thank the many other stroke survivors whose support for this book was most reassuring to me. I am grateful to so many for allowing me to incorporate their words, and I am sorry that I could not include you all.

Finally, I would like to thank the unknown A&E doctor and unknown ward doctor who both chose not to ignore and dismiss my symptoms (apparently it does happen!) and consequently arranged for the brain scan. I will be forever in their debt.

Below are some details about the consultancy I have set up following my stroke. Please do get in touch if you'd like to contact me.

AMCAN Consultancy & Training Ltd

Through AMCAN Consultancy & Training Ltd, Andy McCann is available for speaking engagements, life-coaching, clinical hypnotherapy (including confidence building after stroke), vocational rehabilitation, stress-management courses and the writing and producing of a wide range of tailor-made educational resources.

AMCAN Consultancy & Training Ltd
Suite 142, The Business Centre
61 Wellfield Road
Roath, Cardiff CF24 3DG
www.amcanct.co.uk
Email: andy@amcanct.co.uk

Foreword

My father died of a stroke when he was 52 years of age, my best friend suffered a stroke whilst making breakfast one morning and has made a near full recovery. Yet how many people really know what a stroke is, other than it being a medical term that describes loss of blood flow to a part of the brain? How many of us know about the different types of stroke? Or the at-risk groups, hereditary factors, or lifestyle causes – very few I imagine. Why? Probably because strokes happen to other people and therefore we assume won't happen to us. The reality is strokes do happen to people like us, people like Andy McCann, an active PE teacher who too suffered a stroke. As a result of the stroke Andy set out to learn everything he could about strokes, their causes, the facts and the realities.

In the final analysis we owe it to ourselves to take full responsibility for our health and wellbeing, and the fastest route to understanding is through knowledge. But knowledge alone is not enough, it never has been, it is applied knowledge that is the key to understanding. So if you apply the knowledge you gain from this book, you will reduce the risk of stroke in your life and make the right choices for your wellbeing.

Robin Sieger, author of Natural Born Winners
and Chairman, Sieger International Ltd

Foreword

Someone somewhere within the UK has a stroke every five minutes of every day, every year. It is the third biggest killer and one of the biggest causes of disability across the population. Any stroke is always unexpected as there are very rarely any warning signs that it is about to happen. It is impossible to say why a stroke happens when it does and not at some other time, and equally difficult to say why some people have a stroke and why others do not. All strokes are different. In fact no two are alike. How people are affected and how they recover becomes very individual to that person. So when a stroke happens to someone like Andy McCann, a fit young man, it comes as a great shock both to him and his family.

This book describes Andy's journey through the acute phase of his stroke and through rehabilitation. It gives an account of his experiences and offers some solutions to practical problems. It gives clear explanations of some of the more bewildering medical terms and describes some of the therapies and treatments he received. The book makes very useful reading for anyone affected by stroke, whether as a survivor, carer or family member. Opinions and advice expressed in the book are not, however, always to be taken as expressing the opinions and recommendations of The Stroke Association. They are, quite properly, Andy's.

The Stroke Association's mission is to prevent strokes and reduce their effect through providing services, campaigning, educating and research. We want to see a world where there are fewer strokes and all those touched by stroke get the help they need.

We would like to wish Andy every success with the book.

The Stroke Association (UK)

Introduction

'This year, thousands of families will be thrown into turmoil, threatened by poverty and placed under unbearable strain when their main breadwinner is debilitated by stroke.'

The Stroke Association (UK), personal communication, 2004

The word 'stroke' is incorporated into the everyday use of the English language. It can have many meanings and is used as both noun and verb. Furthermore, it can also be paired with words (e.g. 'sunstroke'). In addition, it is often used in phrases such as 'at the stroke of midnight', 'a stroke of luck', and 'a stroke of genius'. Now, in the 21st century, most people will have also used or heard the phrase '…had a stroke'. For some 300 years this description has been firmly ingrained in the English language to encompass a variety of neurological conditions. In this context, a stroke is actually really a collection of neurological symptoms and signs as an injury to the brain has repercussions throughout the body. Put very simply, a stroke refers to the brain equivalent of a heart attack, and as such is now even referred to as a 'brain attack' by some doctors (see Chapter 6 'What Is a Stroke?').

Unfortunately, in many cases the stroke will end the life of the individual who has had it. For those who survive, and for their families and loved ones, at best life will be suspended, while at worst the quality of life will be severely and permanently affected. The majority of stroke survivors fall somewhere between the two extremes, but what is consistent across all cases is that life will never be the same again.

I have written this book as a result of my unexpected introduction to this neurological 'world of stroke' when I surprised myself, and everyone who knew me, by actually having and surviving one. I was just 37 years of age, a physical education teacher who was physically fit and strong, and in good health.

Having survived the stroke, I had to quickly come to terms with a particularly disagreeable affliction I knew little about, and yet, statistically, should have been far more aware of. I then had to try to recover from it, try to establish why it had happened to me and see what steps I could take to prevent another one. Finally, I had to decide how best to incorporate positively the whole experience into my day-to-day existence, and so be able to continue with the rest of my life.

Even as I lay in hospital during the first days after the stroke, it occurred to me that what unites victims of stroke is simply the term used, and even that is a bit vague and nondescript. In my mind, I instantly labelled myself and became 'someone who had suffered a stroke'. As the months passed by, I needed to find out more about the stroke community that I had become a part of. It is, therefore, as a result of my own experience that I will use the term 'stroke' and not 'brain attack' throughout this book. This is simply because all the medical staff I came into contact with used it with me. However, when discussing the nature of stroke in Chapter 6, I hope to clarify and explain what this term actually means in easily accessible language.

The human body as a whole, and the brain as an organ within the body, are undoubtedly extremely resilient. Factors that contribute to brain damage include infection; exposure to drugs, alcohol and other toxic substances; inadequate nutrition; and, of course, stroke. While some of these may be the result of accidents, many individuals seem to dismiss, quite casually, habits and behaviour that cause damage to their body and brain. In my case, the stroke, and resulting damage to my brain, seems to have been spontaneous without any identifiable external trauma or inadvisable behaviour. However, this is quite unusual as a 'stroke is often an endpoint in a lifetime of accumulated risk' (Wiebers 2001, p.277). This statement makes a very important point, and one I will revisit several times during the book because, despite my own experience, the majority of strokes can be avoided. Nevertheless, whatever the underlying cause of a stroke, the symptoms of brain damage as they relate to stroke are reasonably constant and are outlined in this book through my own experience in Part I, and are then further developed in Part II. However, at the risk of complicating the issue at this stage, I should mention that the symptoms can vary in terms of their severity, as can the damage caused by a stroke, and it is worth stating from the outset that both the immediate and lasting effects of stroke vary from individual to individual.

For those of us unfortunate to suffer a stroke, but fortunate to survive it and be still able to enjoy a good quality of life, the whole experience will undoubtedly remain entirely personal. Every person approaches life and the world around them in a slightly different way, because each person's brain is different. Our individual perspective is first determined by genetics and then moulded by life's many experiences. Through the visual (sight), auditory (hearing), olfactory (smell) and kinaesthetic (tactile) processes, our brain receives external stimuli, which it then generalises, distorts, filters, deletes or saves. As we get older, we assimilate new experiences with old ones. We develop a frame of reference, which we use to assess events and experiences. The result, in the same way that two eyewitnesses may give very different accounts of the same event, is that none of us can feel exactly what another person feels. However, there will always be some common ground and Part II introduces, in some detail, the range of possible effects and prognoses following a stroke.

The greatest medical advances have taken place since the beginning of the 20th century and they have easily surpassed all that was known about stroke in all previous history. Consequently, we are now better informed about stroke than ever before. In order to help you to understand the causes and effects of stroke, Part II invites you to follow a basic, but in my view very necessary, introductory journey into the workings of the brain. This is an aspect of the world of stroke that some people (other than neurosurgeons) may find tedious, but I found absolutely fascinating. After all, as the result of 240 million years of evolution, the human brain is the single most evolved organ ever. To be honest, even though I had some knowledge of some aspects of the functions of the brain in my teaching and sports coaching career, I had previously given little thought to how it has evolved and actually works.

Despite my teaching background, my interest in physical education, and now my experience of stroke, this book is not written as a medical or scientific textbook, though I do use many medical terms associated with stroke that are currently in use. Throughout the centuries, the medical profession seems to have developed a word for every specific neural or mental function for which patients may find themselves partly or wholly deprived, which can be a cause of confusion. These include aphonia, aphemia, aphasia, alexia, apraxia, agnosia, ataxia, diplopia, dysarthria, dysphagia, dyspraxia, and so on (see Glossary for definitions). In addition, other common terms used in stroke cases are 'deficit' and 'loss of function'. As a result, the following phrases will be heard often: a loss of speech, a loss of language, a loss of memory, a loss of vision, a loss of dexterity, and a loss of identity. Therefore, when faced with a combination of both phrases that describe functional deficits, and the specific words used for each, it is easy to end up confused. While an alphabetical glossary of terms is available at the end of the book, an explanation of specialist terminology as it appears will be given in accompanying boxes.

So, as you read through the book, and appreciate a little more how we function as living beings, you will be introduced to the many 'deficits' that may exist due to brain damage as a result of stroke. To help illustrate this, I have included, in Appendix I, some short extracts of stroke survivors' stories, which are reproduced in this book completely unedited, and in their own words. You will discover, through my own experience and the experiences of others, that even though language problems are very commonly associated with stroke, both the cause of such problems and how they affect this critical skill and aspect of human behaviour can vary greatly from case to case. You will soon appreciate that there are other common problems as a result of stroke, including: physical changes (ranging from both fine and gross motor skills to immobility and paralysis); cognitive changes (including slowed thought processing, attention, memory); psychosocial changes (including personality and behaviour); and executive changes (essentially the planning and evaluating of the execution of a given task).

Among well-known examples that illustrate these different problems is that of a senior American judge who caused embarrassment and confusion when he returned to work following a stroke that affected the right side of his brain. The right side of the brain helps us to make judgements, and he became unable to weigh evidence as he had done before the stroke. As a result he is said to have been extremely unperturbed in sentencing minor offenders to life, while allowing the more serious criminals to go free. Meanwhile, another case refers to a man who lost the ability to recognise familiar faces (known as prosopagnosia). His recovery was generally good, but eventually he insisted that his wife wear a ribbon in her hair as on one occasion, after a social function, he attempted to take the wrong woman home. A third case relates the story of a farmer who, each day, was unable to recognise his wife until she actually spoke. It is reported that this inability to recognise faces also extended to his livestock and he repeatedly tried to milk his bull! A further case is that of a man who had great difficulty in controlling his limbs when moving from sitting to standing, or when lifting his arms to wave, and yet he remained able to perform more complex movements, such as removing his glasses from his head.

My own stroke affected the area of the brain known as the cerebellum, the most clearly understood function of which is to co-ordinate and refine body movements. Therefore, people with damage to their cerebellum are usually able to perceive the world normally. I'm told by many who know me that this phrase might not apply to me, rather it should mean simply that I perceive the world in the way that I did before the stroke!

Those of us who survive a cerebellar stroke are fortunate. First, cerebellar strokes are often caused by an emergency relating to the vertebrobasillary arterial system. Simply speaking, this is the system that supplies blood to the clinically important back sections of the brain and anything 'affecting the vertebrobasillary arterial system may cause high morbidity and mortality rate' (Taycan et al. 2002). Second, cerebellar strokes occur in less than 1.5 per cent of stroke patients and as a result are not always identified and treated with the immediate medical attention required in the case of a stroke. Third, the cerebellum is located behind the brainstem (see Chapter 7 'The Brain and Its Blood Supply') and may swell, causing sudden death.

On a personal note, having survived the cerebellar stroke and previously having been a sportsman, self-defence and martial art instructor, and physical education teacher – accepting damage to this area, and having to identify and accept the possible causes and risk factors of further strokes, was very hard. The word perspective took on a far deeper meaning for me than it had previously, and with time, discipline, positive thinking and the support of doctors, therapists, family, friends and my partner, Anne, I was able to move forward. Eventually, as I learned more about strokes and made good progress in terms of my recovery, I became grateful that I was a 'stroke survivor' and refused to be called a 'stroke victim'.

This book began simply as a myriad of private notes written by me for my own benefit. Making notes was an exercise through which I was able to discover what I was actually thinking, feeling and experiencing. Without doing this, I was unable to clarify and organise my thoughts. I had never been one to express my feelings, so my thoughts and feelings were not clear to anyone, including me. Perhaps typically for a teenage boy, I had expended a lot of effort in my adolescent years ensuring that I could effectively disguise my feelings – happiness, fear, gratitude, and even affection. On reflection, I continued with this attitude well into adulthood. Then quite suddenly, having survived the devastation of the early months of 2004, I realised that my disguise had been ripped away from me. I felt broken and vulnerable.

So, by writing down my emotions and an account of what I was experiencing, I gained control over my situation and refused to be overwhelmed and completely engulfed by it. It was only at this time in my recovery that I woke up to the reality of having had a stroke, which was compounded by the obvious lack of understanding that exists in society of this very real killer. I decided to combine the medical advice I received with my knowledge and understanding both of the human body and of Eastern

approaches to health, which I had accumulated in 20 years of practising
martial arts. In so doing, I sought to redevelop my physical capabilities as
much as possible and to establish a new psychological equilibrium, therefore producing a healthy excitement as to what the future may have in store.
The integrated approach that I developed along with the techniques and
therapies (including training professionally as a clinical hypnotherapist)
that I used throughout my recovery are placed in context and explained
fully in Chapter 10 'A Toolkit for Recovery and Prevention'.

I am pleased to have been able to write this book. I sincerely hope that
it will be of interest to you and, depending on why you are reading it, it may
even change how you think about stroke in a variety of ways:

- As you will be able to tell by now, it illustrates my personal
  experiences, which may provide some comfort to others who
  have experienced similar problems.

- It may simply contribute to you developing a greater
  understanding of stroke through the factual information that is
  included (you could take this opportunity to pause and try to
  recall one stroke fact that you have read in this introduction!).
  After all, educating yourself about stroke is a significant step
  towards both prevention and recognising the warning signs and
  symptoms of stroke.

- Some of the practical methods I employed to support my
  recovery may be of interest and benefit to you whether you have
  had a stroke, are at high risk of a stroke, or not – although, they
  should of course be discussed with appropriate carers and
  medical supervisors.

- We live in a world of some financial uncertainty and the need
  for sound financial planning with regard to life insurance,
  healthcare and income protection is more important than ever
  and this may stimulate you to be proactive with regard to such
  things. This area is discussed in Chapter 11 'Financial Matters'.

Whether any of the above applies to you directly or not, what is vital is that
all possible preventive measures associated with stroke are acted upon; that
the symptoms of stroke are more widely recognised; that the simple check
tests for stroke are more widely known; and that the myth of age-related-
ness and stroke is dispelled. To coincide with the World Health Organization's (WHO: see Glossary) release of a definitive atlas of the global heart
disease and stroke epidemic, Dr Robert Beaglehole, the WHO Director of

Chronic Disease and Health Promotion, stated: 'The old stereotype of cardiovascular diseases affecting only stressed, overweight middle-aged men in developed countries no longer applies.' For some individuals, significant steps can be made to recovery and improving quality of life. By paying due attention to these issues it will be possible significantly to reduce the worldwide effects of stroke on individuals, families and society. Due to the nature of strokes, it is easy to feel very alone in the experience. The statistics and facts tell a different story:

- The seriousness of stroke combined with the survival statistics means that stroke is the biggest cause of disability in developed countries.

- Stroke is currently the third largest cause of death after heart disease and cancer in the world.

- Approximately 25 per cent of stroke sufferers die as a result of the stroke or its complications.

- Almost 50 per cent of stroke survivors have moderate to severe health impairments and long-term disabilities.

- In both the UK and Canada, over a quarter of a million are living with long-term disability as a result of stroke.

- Just 26 per cent recover most or all normal health and function after a stroke.

- One recent health survey showed that among adults aged fifty, 97 per cent could not identify a single stroke symptom.

It is clear from the health statistics associated with stroke that many families have a direct association with the syndrome and yet there are relatively few resource books available. Many books, whether they are fiction, non-fiction, or from the self-help genre, are based purely on imagination, or written with second-hand information. This book by contrast is very personal. By definition it has to be; it is largely about me, and my experiences. I do refer to many issues related to stroke, but this book is a unique perspective on the world of stroke as seen through my eyes. It is, therefore, far from a definitive piece of work. The medical information and medical tests contained in this book, along with all described methods of rehabilitation, relate directly to my experience and are not intended for use as a source of medical reference.

Finally, I suppose I would like to have been given time to prepare for what was to come on that January evening in 2004. Of course in an ideal

world I would rather not have had a first-hand experience of stroke. However, the experience has reinforced to me how much a part of other people's
lives my life, my happiness and my health is. It has made me reflect and
appreciate life more, something many people only do when they reach old
age and say, 'I wish I knew then what I know now!' This may come as a surprise to you at this stage of the book, but I have absolutely no doubt that the
rest of my life will be enriched as a result of this experience!

'Life is just one damned thing after another.'

Elbert Hubbard (1856–1915)

Part I

My Stroke: From a Statistic to Personal Discovery

~ Chapter 1 ~

Stroke in Context

'As I have sometimes joked, life comes without an instruction manual – and yet we are born with innate abilities to overcome its challenges.'

Robin Sieger, Natural Born Winners *(2004), p.xiii*

There is a time of significant challenge in everyone's life. A time when faith, values, compassion, patience and pure determination are tested to the limit. At such a time, life itself may seem very unfair. Suffering a stroke is such a time.

Simply speaking, when there is an interruption of blood to part of the heart muscle, an individual suffers what is known as a heart attack; when there is an interruption of blood to part of the brain, an individual suffers what is known as a stroke. In the latter, this disruption of the blood supply results in parts of the brain, which is the most delicate organ in the body, becoming damaged or destroyed. The symptoms of stroke should, therefore, quite clearly have the same alarming significance in being identified that acute chest pain has in identifying a heart attack. In fact, many doctors believe that to have the best chance of limiting damage, strokes should be heeded even more urgently than heart attacks. While I go into much greater detail about the physiology of stroke in Part II, I think that it is worth placing this biological event in context right here, at the beginning of the book.

Every year, some 15 million people suffer a stroke. Generally speaking, one third of people who have an initial stroke die within a year. As a result, stroke is the third leading cause of death in developed countries, behind heart disease and cancer. Talking in figures of millions like this, it becomes very easy to feel remote from the implications, and indeed the reality, of stroke. Perhaps it would be easy to think of it like this: if you are reading this and living in the UK, during the next 60 minutes 12 people will have a stroke. Four of these will recover, four will have permanent disabilities and four will die. If you are living in the US, someone will have a stroke in the time you will take to read this page, and within the last three minutes, while you have opened this book and found your page, someone will have died of a stroke. These 'time/stroke' cycles are constantly repeating 24 hours a day, seven days a week…you will have the idea by now.

Stroke as an 'acquired brain injury'

The neurological syndrome of stroke is actually classified as a non-traumatic brain injury (NTBI) as shown in Figure 1.1.

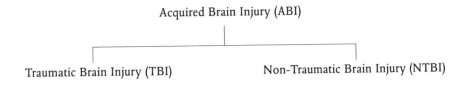

Acquired Brain Injury (ABI)

Traumatic Brain Injury (TBI)   Non-Traumatic Brain Injury (NTBI)

Figure 1.1: The classification of acquired brain injury

This is different from a traumatic brain injury (TBI), which is caused by an 'external energy' or a 'mechanical force'. However, both NTBIs and TBIs come under the general heading of acquired brain injury (ABI). Stated simply, ABI is categorised as occurring after birth and as such is different from a brain injury that is congenital, or the result of a birth trauma, and refers to any damage to the brain caused by an external physical force, or by things of a vascular, degenerative or neurological nature.

- ABI – this is an injury to the brain that is not hereditary, congenital, degenerative or induced by birth trauma. It has occurred after birth.

- TBI – these involve anything that can damage brain tissue and include open or closed head injuries. They may be caused by work-related, domestic, road or sport accidents.

- NTBI – these have more 'indirect' causes, which include stroke and other vascular accidents, tumours, viral infections, metabolic disorders and the inhalation or ingestion of toxic products.

Stroke as a 'disease burden'

While there is no good time to suffer a stroke, many strokes are undoubtedly premature when considered in terms of age. Family, friends and colleagues are all affected by the tragedy. Out of those individuals who have an NTBI caused by stroke each year, a third (an estimated 5.5 million people worldwide) die. Significantly, this leaves almost two thirds surviving. A third of these survivors are left permanently disabled, suffering a range of problems, which affect their quality of life or place in society. The most common of these problems include paralysis of one side of the body and communication difficulties. Stroke is, therefore, quite rightly classified as a major 'disease burden' for society in terms of the 'disability adjusted life years' that are associated with it. Unfortunately, a stroke can lead to a 'life of diminished function and a compromised fulfilment' (Wiebers 2001).

Currently, the US alone spends $30 billion each year in treating stroke. In the UK, the annual stroke-specific costs are estimated to be £2.5 billion. In gross terms, and per head of population, this is obviously less than the US, but it is actually almost twice that spent on coronary heart disease in the UK. This is significant because it makes stroke one of the most expensive conditions to treat. Worse still, the future looks bleak. In terms of being a 'disease burden', stroke is expected to reach a staggering 61 million world-wide by 2020. Despite this prediction (and the increase in death rates and health costs that will inflate as a result) prioritising major stroke issues, such as research and raising awareness of stroke, falls far behind that of other big killers. The UK Stroke Association has highlighted this, reporting that for every £1 spent on stroke research, £20 is spent on heart disease research and £50 is spent on cancer research.

A simple summary of stroke statistics

If you are reading this book, it is likely that you have entered the 'world of stroke' by having one yourself, or knowing someone who has. To continue the theme of placing stroke in context, the statistics below give a rough idea of the scale of the phenomenon.

United Kingdom

- In the United Kingdom someone has a stroke every five minutes.
- Stroke is the UK's third biggest killer.

United States

- In the US someone has a stroke every 45 seconds.
- Every three minutes one of these US stroke victims will die.
- Stroke is the US's third biggest killer.

Canada

- In Canada there are over 50,000 strokes and 16,000 deaths as a result of stroke each year.

Australia

- Over 40,000 Australians suffer stroke each year.
- Stroke is the second biggest killer.

Although 75 to 85 per cent of strokes occur in people over the age of 65, a stroke can occur at any age – even in children. Babies account for one third of strokes in the category of 'new-born to 18-years-of-age' and UK figures illustrate that 10,000 people each year under the age of 55 suffer a stroke. This equates to around 30 per day, over 200 per week. Nevertheless, stroke is uncommon in people who are generally in good health and under 40 years of age. However, at approximately 7pm on Thursday 8 January 2004 I had a stroke, and so contributed directly to the statistics above.

I learned at first hand that there is no discrimination in the people affected by strokes, and many people may not be aware of the high-profile people who have experienced a stroke (see box).

Some famous people who have experienced a stroke

- Winston Churchill – British Prime Minister
- Stan Laurel – English-born comedy writer and actor
- Oliver Hardy – American comedy performer
- Margaret Thatcher – British Prime Minister
- Louis Pasteur – French scientist (developer of rabies vaccine)
- Kirk Douglas – American actor
- Sharon Stone – American actress
- Sir Harry Secombe – Welsh entertainer
- Patricia Neal – American actress
- Luther Vandross – American singer
- Princess Margaret – Member of British Royal Family

~ Chapter 2 ~

My Life Before the Stroke

We all tend to complain about things from time to time. I certainly have done. Like many people, I started to complain and show frustration about more and more trivial things, more and more regularly, as I gradually made my way through my thirties. I am reasonably sure that you will be able to associate your own behaviour with this.

However, my perspectives changed with the stroke. For readers who have not had a stroke, the following exercise may be quite valuable. It is highly likely you have complained about aspects of your life in the past seven days. Think back to what it was that you were unhappy about, and that you spent time and energy on complaining about. Now, imagine that you have suddenly lost everything – your home, your income, even your health. You have lost the ability to move and to speak, and possibly all your dreams for the future. You may never take the dream holiday you have been saving for. You may never see your children grow up. You may never get to meet your grandchildren. You may never get to settle and make good after the argument with your friend or loved one.

Dwell on these thoughts for a short time as they apply to you. Imagine yourself lying or sitting in a room, on your own, with these thoughts. Now, think how you would feel if you suddenly had your life back again! Feel the relief and even joy of simply having what you have now, which may even include gratefully accepting the issue that you remembered complaining about a moment ago. Going through this exercise may even provide you with a new outlook, meaning that if you had to, you would even accept your health not being quite back to what it was.

While this cannot duplicate the feelings and emotions associated with stroke (or many other serious health problems), it does illustrate the need for us all to sometimes spend time appreciating what we have got. Thinking like this certainly helped me to deal with, not just my stroke as a major life event, but how best to reorganise my life and future. I hope that this book will reinforce this idea throughout, but more importantly, illustrate the fact that it is not what happens to you that matters, rather it's what you do about it that counts.

I have included the following brief description of my life simply to illustrate that prior to my stroke I had been confident and active, and with no identifiable health risk factors or warning of what was to come. I was typical of many millions of adults in developed countries. I had a normal life in many ways. I had a good job, a mortgage, a car loan, a bank overdraft (access to many credit cards), bills to pay and the rest of my life to pay them. I combined my career with plenty of other interests. I was successful, very confident, and happily riding along on the wave of life.

I was born just outside London in 1966. Within a few months my parents and I moved to South Wales, where I have lived ever since. It was in Wales that my mother was born and raised, and where she had met my father in 1961 when they were both student teachers of physical education, at Cardiff Teacher Training College. After I completed my primary education, we moved a short distance and settled in the Welsh capital, Cardiff. I was brought up a Roman Catholic and attended a Catholic high school. After high school I remained in Cardiff to continue my studies at college and university. Through my love of sport, I came to study at the same educational institution where my parents had met. In 1985 I began my degree in human movement studies. By this time Cardiff Teacher Training College had been renamed (it is now called the University of Wales Institute, Cardiff) and, along with Loughborough University, was recognised as one of the top specialist sports institutions in the UK.

Before gaining my place at university I was an active teenager and won my school's Victor Ludorum three years running. I swam competitively, which meant my parents had to take me swimming training around five times a week. I played rugby, which involved evening training and weekend games. In addition, I was a member of a tennis club, a badminton club and a golf club. In 1982, aged 17 years and seeking a new and additional challenge, I enrolled in a tang soo do, Korean karate class at the National Sports Centre for Wales, in Cardiff. During my first lesson with a fierce Asian instructor, I knew that I would not stop training until I reached the coveted black belt. This was not because I thought I was particularly good, just that I had set myself that goal. On reflection, prior to my stroke I generally tended to reach the goals that I set myself (largely through hard work rather than natural talent!). This attitude was something useful that was passed down in my genes from my father, an equally determined character. The training was tough and I loved it. Actually, one of the reasons that I did not want to leave Cardiff to study at a different university was that I wanted to continue training at the same karate club. Eventually, out of the 50 or so who started karate in the same class as me, two of us successfully passed the black belt test around five years later, in 1987. For this test, I travelled to Atlanta, Georgia, and was examined by several of the top instructors from around the world.

In my twenties, and while training for the black belt, I developed into quite an aggressive sportsman and set high standards for myself. As well as the university activities such as gymnastics, trampolining, canoeing and athletics, I continued to play rugby and was also training and competing in a variety of martial art competitions. I applied myself to my endeavours fully, and in my third year at university was awarded the prestigious Sports Personality of the Year award. At a sports specialist institution this is something to be proud of and I was given the award over more well-known sportsmen and women including international rugby players and Commonwealth Games participants.

By the time I left full-time education in 1989, with a degree and a post-graduate physical education teaching certificate (PGCE), participating in sport, exercise and physical activity was an integral part of my daily routine. I instructed at my own karate club on a Monday evening; trained at my instructor's club on a Tuesday; instructed at my club on a Wednesday; went rugby training on a Thursday; played squash on a Friday; went to a friend's karate club on a Saturday morning; and played rugby on a Saturday afternoon. I kept Sunday as a rest day. I only played golf! I followed the principle attributed to 83-year-old Mavis Layrer: 'Life's journey is not to arrive at the grave safely, in a well preserved body, but rather to skid in sideways, totally worn out, shouting "Holy shit, what a ride!"'

When I left university, I was lucky enough to be offered a professional karate instructor position in the USA. This was despite the near breakdown of the contract negotiations after my mother had head-butted my instructor (and sponsor) on one of his UK visits. I was his designated chauffeur for the duration of his stay and was extremely busy for the week. My mother attended one of the functions and he wanted to be introduced to her. As they shook hands my instructor bowed his head. Instinctively, but unlike many Western women, so too did my mother, much to his surprise! Bone hit bone. Skull hit skull. I stood there in shock, gradually coming to terms

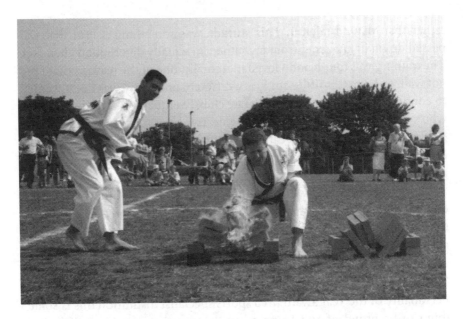

Me breaking some concrete blocks (in an attempt to show off, they are on fire for added effect)

with the fact that my mother had just head-butted my karate instructor. I thought he took it well and was very dignified throughout. I briefly questioned myself as to the effectiveness of his 30 years' martial arts training when the opponent was the youngest of nine children from a Welsh mining town!

Unfortunately, the physical training I was putting my body through left me with a chronic lower back injury, which could have proved problematic for a professional karate instructor. So, after much consideration, and even after a successful minor operation to rectify the problem, I decided to remain in the UK, opting for the financial security of a career as a secondary school physical education teacher. I was extremely lucky. I still wanted to live in Cardiff and was successful in my first application, which was for the position of a boys' physical education teacher in the South Wales valley town of Pontypridd. In 1989 I began teaching at Cardinal Newman Roman Catholic School.

It was during my first year teaching that I experienced what was to become my second sporting love after martial arts – skiing. In truth, I had exaggerated my competence (having never skied!) in order to join the ski trip that first year. Fortunately for me, my early enthusiasm, combined with an astonishing ability to recover my skis quickly after falling, meant that I did not hold back the group and I progressed quickly. So, after a couple of seasons and several trips later, I had become an advanced, aggressive and fearless skier. Skiing was always an experience I enjoyed. Over the years, and as I became more proficient, I was fortunate to ski in Europe, Canada and the USA in many of the world's top resorts. I enjoyed testing my physical capabilities against the elements in the mountains. I liked to be first on the slopes and last off. Consequently, I skied on piste and off piste; in sunshine and in blizzards; in the warm mountain air of the Alps, and in the cold mountain temperatures of Quebec (−45°!).

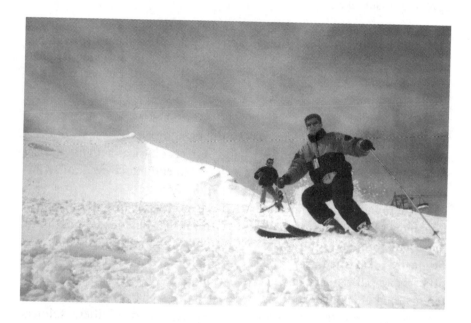

Me skiing in the Alps

My body seemed to cope with the demands that I still continued to put it under reasonably well. However, in 1993, the effects of a rugby injury combined with continuous gymnastic coaching and martial art training left me with a prolapsed cervical disc. I was aware from a sports injuries course that I had followed in university that most neck pain is due to degenerative changes that occur in the invertebral discs of the cervical spine. The concern is always that such degenerative changes in the cervical spine may lead to a very serious condition where there is too much pressure on the spinal cord. When this condition occurs, the entire spinal cord is in danger. I knew that my injury was serious as the pain in my arm and hand, through my chest and down my back was unbearable. Communication between my physiotherapist and my GP resulted in an examination with a consultant surgeon who, following magnetic resonance imaging (MRI: see Glossary), advocated immediate surgery. I did not have to think long about whether to have the operation, known as a *cervical laminectomy*. This was despite the fact that in the worst case unsuccessful surgery would have left me paralysed from the neck down. Ironically, one of the other risk factors associated with the surgical procedure is actually stroke. As I say, the pain and immobility that I suffered at that time was quite unbearable, so I ended up agreeing to surgery.

Cervical laminectomy is derived from cervical (neck) plus lamina (part of the spinal canal's bony structure) and -ectomy (removal). The operation is commonly performed to remove an invertebral disc protrusion or to decompress a nerve root.

The operation was a complete success: the pressure on the spinal cord was released and within six months I had resumed physical activity and set myself the goal of competing in a duathlon (an endurance event of swimming and running) to help with my rehabilitation.

I continued training in the martial arts even after this second spinal operation. However, I increased my interest in self-defence training in its most pure form and joined a specialist jujutsu training group, which was originally established as a resource for high-grade martial artists, police officers and self-defence instructors. Through this, I was exposed to a different group of people and soon appreciated that some of the World War II soldiers were the true self-protection experts. Many of these soldiers trained in the method taught by Captain W.E. Fairbairn, who is largely recognised as having developed the first scientifically researched fighting system in the 1920s, while he was Assistant Commissioner of the Shanghai Municipal Police. Such techniques, and the mindset needed to survive a violent encounter, had been proven time and time again in the most testing of circumstances.

Eventually I became an instructor with the group and became involved in teaching self-protection instructors how to teach, and what to teach. I felt honoured when a former member of the elite Royal Marine Commandos, whose specialist duties had included time in Ireland and royal protection for the Duke of Edinburgh, told me that training with me was the most painful and useful self-protection session he had ever done.

Still teaching full-time in school, I eventually reached high grades and achieved black belts and internationally recognised instructor certificates in more than one fighting discipline. For two years, I travelled to the USA to train exclusively with Professor Tom Muncy, one of the world's leading instructors in the martial art of torite jutsu – the application of pressure points to the martial arts (for both combat and health). In the four years leading up to the start of 2004 (when I had the stroke) I gained a black belt in torite jutsu; passed a fourth degree black belt test in my original discipline of tang soo do karate; passed an additional advanced test and was awarded the title of 'Martial Art Master'; was voted 'Master Instructor of the Year' by Dragon Black Belt Academy International for my martial arts teaching skills; and was given a British National Martial Arts Association award in recognition of my outstanding contribution to martial arts in the UK. A common phrase used by self-defence instructors is that 'courage is simply understanding that you are afraid, yet still managing to operate effectively'. This outlook was one I strived to adhere to following my unexpected stroke.

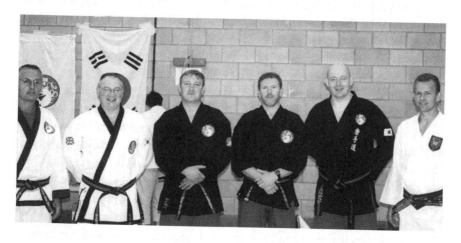

Me at the 2002 British Championships with fellow national instructors from Scotland and England (I am third from right)

As well as seeking physical challenges, I also enjoyed the challenges that my teaching career brought. I successfully completed an MA (Ed) while still working full-time and, as with my first karate class, witnessed many colleagues on the course give up due to the demands placed upon them. Following a promotion, I was appointed Head of Physical Education and led the PE department to winning the 1998 Midland Bank Welsh National

School Sports Award for all-round excellence. As a coach I was also success-ful. My boys' gymnastic team won Welsh titles on three occasions and my senior rugby team, coached by myself and my friend Gerry McLoughlin (a former Irish and British Lion prop forward), won the Welsh Rugby Union's U-19 Cup at the Millennium Stadium in Cardiff. Rugby is extremely popu-lar in Wales, and the president of my school's rugby district stated that our cup win was the most 'momentous achievement in the 100 year history of the district'. In addition, my colleagues in the PE department and I achieved great success through our pupils' performance in external examinations every year.

As I became more experienced, I was soon invited to run courses for physical education student teachers at my former university, and facilitate courses for practising teachers of physical education through the county advisory service. I thought nothing of speaking in front of large, educated audiences and meeting, head on, the challenges that such a task brings. In fact, I was frequently told, by colleagues and friends, that I always dis-played a calm and confident manner in the most trying of circumstances.

The years passed by, and professional opportunities within the school became available. I became a Head of Year, Head of Post 16 Education and, eventually, Assistant Headteacher. I worked no harder than many of my colleagues, or people in other professions, but the pace of my day was fran-tic and the length of my working days increased.

On reflection, I suppose I spent over 20 years creating an image for myself of invulnerability. As it transpired on that day in January 2004, I was sadly mistaken. In my mind, I was both physically invulnerable and emo-tionally strong. I was also healthy. I had watched my alcohol intake for years (after the usual drinking expected as a student!); I did not smoke; I did not think that I let the stress of work upset me, and was even at times a calm-ing influence on others around me; and I had lots of interests.

I started to spend more time with a colleague, Anne, outside of work. Anne had joined the teaching staff some years after me and we became friends. Eventually, and after much persuasion from me, she agreed that we would go out together. This relationship seemed to work and we did not really see each other much in work due to the pace of the teaching day. I moved into Anne's house a few years later and in 2002 we bought a house together.

Like most of us busily struggling through the daily routine of life, I gave very little thought to stroke through all these years. I believed that heart disease and cancer were the things to watch out for! I thought this, despite coming into contact with stroke survivors on several occasions over a period of 30 years. My first introduction to a stroke victim came when I was a child. My grandfather, known as 'Mac', had a great friend, Mr Mitchell, known as 'Mitch'. When I was about eight years of age, I am ashamed to say I found 'Mitch' quite scary. He was tall, but it wasn't his size that scared me, it was the patch over the eye on the droopy side of his face and his shuffle that really scared me. 'Mitch' was a stroke survivor, but as a boy I used to simply think that he wasn't normal.

I was still young when I had my second introduction to a stroke victim – my father's uncle, Mike. To me, Uncle Mike was a little different to 'Mitch'. I knew him well before he had a stroke; before his face dropped on one side; before he had problems speaking and remembering words; and before he kept calling me a 'good girl'. Uncle Mike had developed, as do many stroke sufferers, confusion with words. However, as a ten-year-old who was used to playing cricket and soccer with him in the garden, this change in him was difficult to cope with. The first time he called me a 'good girl', I must have been around ten years old. I stood with my mouth open, looking around the room for support from my parents and Uncle Mike's wife, Aunty Rita. None came. I remember thinking, have they all gone mad? I haven't come here visiting him to be called a 'good girl'. Nevertheless, at the time something stopped me making a fuss and I just accepted it. 'He's a good girl,' Uncle Mike repeated as he sat in his chair and pinched my knee.

'Uncle Mike gets confused with words since his stroke,' I was told as we drove home.

'Yes, but he doesn't think I am a girl does he?' I needed reassurance and did not even ask what a stroke was.

'No, it's just he uses the wrong words sometimes. He knows you're still a boy.'

As a ten-year-old boy, I wasn't convinced!

My third encounter with a stroke victim was far more recent when an elderly uncle of mine had a stroke. This happened just a few years ago, while he and my aunt were on holiday in Tenerife. Unfortunately, he has been confined to a wheelchair ever since, with the left side of his body being affected. When I visited him, first in hospital and then at home, I certainly did not think that the next person I would know to suffer stroke was going to be me. However, in 2004 my stroke intruded upon my life. For some people, the onset and symptoms of stroke are subtle – very unlike the pain of a heart attack. For me it was not so subtle – it was spontaneous, debilitating and frightening. It was 8 January 2004, and I was just 37 years old.

~ Chapter 3 ~

My Life Changes

'In February 1965 Stan had another stroke, and by 23rd February it became clear that he would not recover. As he lay in bed, he beckoned to a nurse. "I'd rather be skiing than doing this," he murmured. "Do you ski Mr Laurel?" said the nurse.

"No," said Stan, "but I'd rather be doing that than this." A few minutes later he was dead.'

Neil Grant, Laurel & Hardy: Quote Unquote *(1994), p.79*

The first few days

It was early in the morning and I had just spent my second night in hospital. I had been sleeping from early the previous evening and had slept uninterrupted throughout the night. I must have been sleeping for around 15 hours when I was woken by a ward nurse, who was accompanied by one of the many doctors I had seen the day before. They told me that it was Saturday morning. To be honest, that did not really seem to mean anything. The hour, date or day seemed irrelevant. The doctor sat down on my bed, which I took as not being a good sign. She told me that she had news I should hear.

'We've had your CT results, Andrew.' My full Christian name appears on medical records. Without pausing, she added, 'I have to tell you that you've had a stroke caused by a blood clot at the brain.'

I lay, silent. You only need to be told something like that once.

A stroke!

I thought back to when the paramedics had arrived about 40 hours earlier. Due to the speech problems I had developed, I knew that the symptoms were that of stroke but didn't really believe that it could have happened to me. I wasn't old. I had barely reached middle age.

A stroke!

I didn't want to believe that something this serious had happened, and was happening to me. I felt that in terms of how I conducted my lifestyle, I had been doing many things right in order to lead a healthy life.

I lay silent after the doctor and nurse had left.

A stroke!

I thought of my grandfather's friend 'Mitch' for the first time in over 20 years. He was over 70 when he had a stroke. I thought of my father's Uncle Mike. He was also over 70 when he had his stroke. I thought of my Uncle Elvet, in his wheelchair, and remembered that he was almost 80 when he had his stroke. It may seem odd, but I thought too of Kirk Douglas, who I knew was exactly 80 when he had his stroke.

Amongst my general state of confusion, I must have been thinking these thoughts for a couple of hours when they were suddenly interrupted, by two of the patients I had met the day before, talking on the bed next to mine.

'You know "Dai Thin", from Maerdy?' said Frank.

'No,' said Ken, 'but I know a "Dai Fat" from Maerdy.'

'That's him, same fella!' Frank insisted. 'He lost 10 stone in weight some years ago!'

Hearing this, I managed an internal smile and tried to put the news in perspective. As I lay there, confined to bed and listening to the conversation next to me, I thought back to a programme I had once seen on the Discovery Channel about expeditions in the frozen ice of the Arctic. A man could be walking over a solid glacier when suddenly the ice would shift and shatter. The result, a whole new landscape would be forced into place. The ice became undulating where it had been flat and huge ravines formed all around him. Due to the tremendous stress in the floes, a whole new world was formed in the time it took him to take one step. As I lay in my hospital bed, I felt like the Arctic explorer. My world had changed and it seemed to happen in the time it took to take one step. I felt stranded and isolated. In truth, I was neither, and was in fact in the best place I could be. Along with Frank and Ken, I was in the Cardiac Ward of the Royal Glamorgan Hospital, Llantrisant, on the edge of the Rhondda Valley, South Wales. A notable difference, however, was that Frank and Ken were both over 65 years of age.

Again, their conversation interrupted my thoughts.

'He could drink beer!' said Frank. 'Before he lost all the weight.'

'Aye, that's for sure,' Ken affirmed. 'He was a big drinker.'

Ken was in his sixties and in the bed next to me. A retired miner, a former biker, he was softly spoken and, to me, seemed to be the quiet, strong type. He had shattered his left leg in 1962 in a motorbike accident and walked with the aid of a stick. Ken explained to me during our first conversation that his daughter and grandchildren said he would never say with five words what he could say with twenty, and asked that I be patient when talking to him. Luckily for him, I wasn't going anywhere, and ironically 'patient' is a term that applied directly to me. During my time in the Royal Glamorgan Hospital, we had many hours of conversations, with Ken doing most of the talking, and his daughter and grandchildren were certainly right. Nevertheless, he was a real source of encouragement to me throughout that first week.

Frank was in the bed opposite me and to the left. Frank was 71 and lived with his sister. Frank was the first person I communicated with on the ward when I regained a degree of consciousness the day before, which was my first morning on the ward. I didn't have much choice at the time, as when I had opened my eyes, he was sitting on my bed grinning, with a mouth full of what seemed like unusually white dentures.

'You came in at four o'clock this morning, but you probably don't remember,' Frank had said, seeming happy to fill in the gaps that he thought I might have in my mind. 'You didn't disturb us much, so don't worry about it.'

Talking to him for the first time, I could not have cared less whether I had caused a huge disturbance when I had arrived. However, Frank was right about me being disorientated. I should have been on my way to work that morning in the same way as I had done every Friday morning for 15 years. Instead, I was lying on a hospital bed with little inclination to do anything and too weak to move. My head hurt very badly. My eyes were difficult to move, straining and throbbing in the light. My limbs felt strange, as if unattached to my body. When I looked down along my body and legs towards my feet, I realised that I was still wearing the clothes that I was wearing when the ambulance arrived for me the night before.

On my upper body, I had on a grey T-shirt. I remembered that it was a present from the owner of the hotel where I had stayed in the Pyrenees on a ski trip with 42 schoolchildren, just three weeks earlier. On my legs, I had on a pair of loose, black, karate training trousers, which I had also been wearing the evening before. My feet were without socks. Then I remembered. I had been teaching a class – my clothes made up the training kit that I was wearing. I looked again and realised that I was covered in vomit. A memory of travelling by ambulance came into my head. Then I realised that there was something even worse than being covered in sick and wearing sweaty, smelly clothes. It was an emotion. It was an emotion that I had rarely experienced. I was very scared!

On the Thursday evening, completely unaware that I was soon to be admitted to hospital, I was in the gym as usual. I had been looking forward to training, or at least instructing at the jujutsu club, all week. We had not been together for three weeks, due to the time of year. Christmas and New Year had quickly followed the ski trip I had been on. A period of the year that is good fun for most people, but with my enthusiasm for 'fighting' (as Anne called it) I always found that it interrupted the routine of training. As had become usual in recent years, I ran the session.

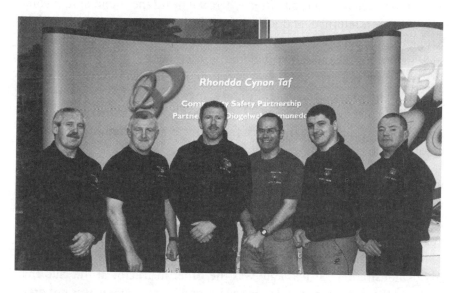

Me with some of my regular jujutsu training partners and fellow instructors (I am third from left, and Paul and Mark are on my right and left respectively)

I had planned a session that would not be physically demanding. We had probably all over-indulged on food and drink during the festive period. In fact, during the warm-up, Ceri, one of the smallest and most experienced members of the club, proudly stated that he had put on half a stone over the two weeks of the Christmas period. Towards the end of the year, Ceri had become the club's self-appointed chief recruiter, often bringing with him a guest from the pubs and clubs in the town. Several were doormen, and, as is usual with doormen, they were often large and looked intimidating. Unfortunately, a flaw in Ceri's recruitment campaign was that they tended to experience too much pain, always by his hand (or knee, or head, or throw, or arm lock!), and none lasted more than a couple of sessions. Paul, one of the other instructors, announced he had started attending Weight Watchers the night before. A more important reason for an easy night's training for me personally was that I had told Anne that I would only instruct that session. Several nights earlier, a 'pop' in the back of my head woke me up and I had subsequently become aware of a stiff neck and an annoying headache that I seemed unable to shake off.

As I conducted the warm-up, I reminded the group that Paul was the first to throw up during training following the Christmas break the year before. We all remembered that he had discreetly left the training hall and gone into the changing room, from where we heard the sound of him vomiting. He soon returned, and joined in with the training as if nothing had happened. I would often tell Anne stories like this, and she always found such behaviour incomprehensible from grown men.

'Why do you put yourselves through it?' she would ask. She just laughed when I gave the usual fighter's answer, 'The harder you train to fight, the easier the fight!' I could never really answer the question as I hoped never actually to end up in a fight! It was just something that we all enjoyed doing.

So, on this occasion I announced to the group, thinking that Anne would be proud of my newfound maturity, 'We're all another year older. It's now 2004. Despite the year's training, we're all probably less fit than a year ago. We will have a quiet evening and ease ourselves gently into training this year.'

I put each member of the class together with a partner, choosing Paul as my demonstration partner. Paul was the other instructor at the club that night, as Brian, another regular instructor and hulk of a man, was not present. Paul and I ran the junior section together. Paul, a hard man, had been in the army and the Metropolitan Police as a physical training instructor. In the mid-1990s, he transferred to South Wales Police, and his children attended the school where I taught. A police instructor for handcuffs, baton, gas, first aid and public order, Paul is a black belt in jujutsu and a reasonable boxer. His real strength, however, has always been that he fights like a rabid dog. After many years of training together, I am still unsure as to whether all the fingers in my eyes, elbows in my nose, scram marks over my body that I received from him were accidental or not. I would arrive home and Anne would ask again, 'And why do you do it?' I also chose Paul because he liked to work at slow instructional speed at times. With it being the first session after the Christmas break, and after him throwing up last year, I knew that this would be one of them. So the very last thing I expected that night was to be rushed from the gym in an ambulance.

As Frank continued to sit on my bed that first Friday morning, he asked me, 'What are you in here for, Andrew?'

Frank seemed completely at home on the hospital ward and glad of the company. He was even aware enough to remember my name from the nurses who had admitted me to the ward in the middle of the night, four hours earlier.

'I don't know,' I was able to mumble slowly, taking time over the pronunciation of each word and very glad that I could speak. At that time I was clinging on to one diagnosis suggested to me in the Accident and Emergency (A&E) room, and so I added, 'Perhaps a migraine?'

'Oh!' Frank appeared disappointed that it was nothing worse and seemed genuinely excited when he said, 'They'll do lots of tests. You'll be well looked after here. They'll find out what's happened to you, all right. Do you want a sweet?'

I declined the offer of a sweet and just lay there. My head really did hurt. Altogether I was experiencing a strange feeling. I knew of the hospital that I was in, but didn't know where it was situated, since it had recently been built. Consequently, I did not know where I was in relation to towns or villages. Somewhat strangely, I almost felt like I was on a holiday and things were not much different to lying in a hotel room in another, faraway country. I lay there feeling completely detached from the world I knew. Once again, I thought back to the events of the previous evening and to the paramedics arriving at the gym.

By the time the paramedics arrived I was trying to sit upright on the floor and was fighting the feeling that I was falling off it. I had a severe case of *vertigo*. In addition, I was nauseous and throwing up and had lost all muscular control. My face, mouth and throat were paralysed, and I was unable to move.

As the group had been working out, I realised that I did not feel quite right. I told Paul that I felt unwell and was going to the side to sit down. As I finished speaking, I was instantly struck with the worst case of dizziness I have ever experienced and I tried to lower myself to the floor in order to cope with it. I could not stand, let alone walk. When safely on the floor I started to sway and lost the ability to focus, developing double vision. The first time I vomited, I was taken by surprise and was sick down the front of my T-shirt, with some of it reaching my trousers. Paul acted fairly swiftly and took control of the situation. He cleared the gym of people, leaving just

Vertigo is defined as an affliction of the head in which objects, though stationary, appear to move in various directions, and the person affected finds it difficult to maintain an erect posture. It is often accompanied by nausea and occasionally vomiting and is generally worsened by motion. Sometimes caused by blood vessel compression of balance nerves.

Mark, another instructor, and him looking after me. Within seconds I had become a heaving, helpless, weak wreck that was unable to move. I had been transformed from a fit, athletic physical education teacher and martial art instructor instantly – or to use a more appropriate term, at a stroke.

Mark quickly decided to get me a bowl (actually it was a waste paper bin), as the vomiting was, by that time, almost continuous. I had lost the ability both to talk and to swallow. While the ability to talk may not (as was once thought) be the crucial factor that distinguishes humans from animals, losing the power to talk is definitely one of the most distressing things that can happen to a human being. I lay, groaning and dribbling as I tried to communicate. I could barely see by this stage and closing my eyes eased the discomfort slightly. My head felt as if it was spinning incredibly quickly, whether my eyes were open or closed. That sensation was more extreme than I had ever felt before, and I had been on some crazy fairground rides, performed gymnastics and trampolining routines, and been tossed around in heavy surf by the sea many times. Despite feeling so bad, I remember that I was worried about Mark. Seeing me like this was upsetting him. Paul, too, obviously felt the same about him, because after Mark had passed me the bowl, Paul sent him outside to wait for the ambulance that he had just telephoned for. This did make sense as some months later, Mark told me that, several years before, he had been with his father as he died through the effects of a major stroke.

In contrast to how I felt about Mark, I was not worried about Paul in the slightest. He had seen far worse than this in his professional life, and I knew he had a strange obsession with the unusual – especially where health, bodies and death was concerned. I knew, too, that Paul would be able to remain detached from what was happening to me, and knowing that somehow eased the burden I already felt my condition was having on others.

While we were waiting for the paramedics, Paul decided to phone Anne, to tell her I was unwell. For an instant, the worry of what was happening to me, and whether Mark was coping, left me. Instead, I worried about what Anne was going to say to me, as she had not wanted me to attend the session at all that night. In truth, as I hadn't actually been exerting myself physically I couldn't understand why I was feeling so bad. It is likely that at that time I was going through what is sometimes described as *depersonalisation, de-realisation* or *dissociation*.

Depersonalisation is the experience of oneself not being real, of one's body being alien, of being an onlooker in relation to one's body (often occurring with de-realisation).

De-realisation is a sense of the world being unreal (often occurring with de-personalisation).

Dissociation is a mental response that diverts consciousness from painful or traumatic events.

Throughout all that was happening, I did manage to remain conscious. I was grounded in myself and my understanding of the environment around me was unaffected, but I was unsure of myself in relation to all that was happening. In isolation, this in itself would have been quite disturbing, but due to the physical disorientation, it was a surprisingly protective feeling, and psychologists believe that it may have evolved in humans as a survival mechanism.

As I struggled to remain conscious, and was dwelling on this strange sensation, the first paramedic walked in with Mark. I wanted to suggest that they also check Mark over as he looked so grey, but I couldn't speak.

'What's happened, then?' the paramedic asked.

I dribbled in response.

I knew that I should give him more information to work with, so I attempted to point at my head. My arm was too heavy to lift, and I had no real feeling in it below the elbow.

'A bump on the head, perhaps?' the paramedic asked.

I tried to open my eyes and move my head. Nothing worked. Earlier that day I had addressed an assembly of some 120 18-year-old students, and now I was unable to say simple words.

Paul explained that I had not had a bump on the head and that I had suddenly said that I needed to sit down for a few minutes, as I was feeling dizzy. He described that I soon began complaining of a headache, and before long had started throwing up.

'When did his speech go?' Paul was asked.

'About 20 minutes ago,' he replied.

'We'll just check your blood pressure and heart rate,' said the second paramedic as he slid the rubber cuff up to my upper arm. I dribbled some more as I tried to acknowledge him.

I felt the *blood pressure* monitor's cuff tighten around my biceps, make a noise then slowly begin to deflate. On the beep some seconds later, I could not open my left eye but I forced my right eye open. I was just able to make out one number on the monitor. It said 72. I remember having the clarity of mind to think that that must have been my *heart rate*, and feeling that it was very good, considering the circumstances. I could not, however, keep my eye open long enough to read the blood pressure reading.

Blood pressure (BP) is defined as the pressure exerted by the blood against the walls of the blood vessels, especially the arteries. It varies with the strength of the heartbeat, the elasticity of the arterial walls, the volume and viscosity of the blood, and a person's health, age and physical condition. *Systolic BP* is the blood pressure during the contraction of the left ventricle of the heart. *Diastolic BP* is the blood pressure after the contraction of the heart while the chambers of the heart refill with blood.

Heart rate is defined as the number of beats the heart makes in one minute.

'Your blood pressure reading is fine,' said the paramedic. 'That should rule out the first thing we should be concerned about. You know what that is, don't you?'

I grunted my acknowledgement. I was relieved at the time because I had started to think that I was having a stroke. In fact, later on in A&E, the paramedic told Anne's sister that I probably had some sort of viral flu.

After being wheeled out of the gym on an ambulance stretcher, I had an uncomfortable journey in the ambulance. The oxygen I was given helped slightly and the paramedic obliged me by pulling the mask off in time for me to throw up at frequent intervals. Unfortunately, as I was also unable to swallow I frequently started choking on my own vomit. The paramedic helped to clear my airway, sat me up slightly and spoke confidently. He made the same idle conversation that most people make with teachers, 'Teacher, eh? I couldn't do your job. It would be all right if it wasn't for the kids!'

Having arrived at the hospital, the paramedics wheeled me into a consultation room. I was lucky the hospital was having a quiet night. I have since heard that one person who was eventually found to have had a stroke was actually mugged in an A&E department while he was waiting to be examined. Apparently, in some areas of the country gangs actively target A&E units in order to find even more vulnerable victims. If I had been targeted in this way, I would quite literally have been unable to move or shout for help.

When I was safely in the consultation room, the trolley I was on rattled loudly as by now my whole body was shaking uncontrollably. I had lost all control and was still unable to speak. The consultation room was spinning as much as the gym had been earlier, and I continued to throw up. By now this was really very unpleasant and consisted only of black bile. My head was hurting worse than I had ever known and I could not really see. A doctor and nurse were with me straight away and they seemed to take a moment to observe what they had in front of them. They saw a sweaty male, wearing a pair of karate training trousers and covered in vomit, shaking from his head down to his toes while heaving loudly. Making an unnecessary amount of noise while being sick, according to my mother, is apparently something passed down in my genes from my father. I have told him since the stroke that I would have preferred something useful, like do-it-yourself skills or an understanding of car maintenance!

The nurse attached a new *sphygmomanometer* to my right bicep and switched it on. This was my first experience of an automatic blood pressure (BP) machine. I did not know then how familiar they would become to me over the following months. It inflated automatically and then deflated over a period of seconds. It provided her with my systolic and diastolic BP readings, my heart rate and a blood *oxygen saturation* analysis. Then she attached pads to my chest and connected me to an *electrocardiogram* (ECG) machine, which bleeped continuously, and she shone an *ophthalmoscope* into my eyes.

Paul and Mark, having followed in a car, were outside and had briefed the doctor as to the symptoms I had shown in the gym. Fortunately, the doctor decided to give me an injection, probably an *antiemetic*, to help with the vomiting. It was given in the muscle of my right leg. I decided to try to speak but still had little control over my jaw, lips and tongue. I did not know it at the time, but my *cranial nerves* were being affected. The doctor and nurse both asked me questions. I was relieved that I understood the questions, and consequently tried in vain to make myself understood. I was confused by the fact that I was able to understand language but not able to speak.

I had been in the consultation room about an hour before the doctor told me that Anne was outside. By that time I was connected to several machines, all bleeping at various intervals. Fortunately, the injection had

Sphygmomanometer is a blood pressure monitor.

Oxygen saturation is the percentage of haemoglobin (the oxygen-carrying part of the red blood cell) that is carrying oxygen. (See also Glossary.)

Electrocardiogram (ECG) is generally used in the investigation of heart disease or simply to monitor heart rate. It is capable of recording the electrical activity of the heart from electrodes placed on the skin in specific locations around the torso. The ECGs of today are compact, lightweight and placed on trolleys, which can be wheeled to any location in the hospital.

Ophthalmoscope is a pen-like device that allows doctors to check for any abnormal eye movements, eye reflexes or swelling of the brain through an examination of the capillaries at the back of the eyes. If the brain is under high pressure, there is generally a swelling of the optic nerve.

Antiemetic is a drug used to prevent nausea and vomiting.

Cranial nerves control the sensory and muscle functions around the eyes, face and throat. There are two sets each of 12 cranial nerves. Each set involves one side of the body.

the desired effect and I had stopped heaving so regularly. However, my body had gone into spasm and I still could not speak.

'Your partner is outside, shall I show her in?' asked the doctor.

I managed to move my head slightly and I was able to indicate that I didn't want to see her at that time. I was naïve enough about my condition to be determined to be able to speak at least a little when I was eventually to see Anne. I couldn't bear causing her more distress than she was already going to have when she first saw me. The doctor understood and did not try to persuade me to let her in. So there we stayed, Anne on the outside and me lying on the hospital trolley, concentrating on trying to regain control of my tongue.

As I lay there, I remembered a recent interview with Kirk Douglas I had seen on BBC's *Parkinson* show. I had always enjoyed Kirk Douglas films, particularly the Westerns. Kirk had suffered a stroke in 1995, which left him unable to speak for some time. Seeing him being interviewed by Michael Parkinson after his stroke I remembered being moved and thinking that he was every bit as tough in real life as the characters he played in his films. As I lay there, and though I didn't know yet that my speech impairment was, like Kirk Douglas's, caused by a stroke, I had the presence of mind to try to remember what exercises he said he had done with his speech therapist. I seemed to remember he was encouraged to loosen his

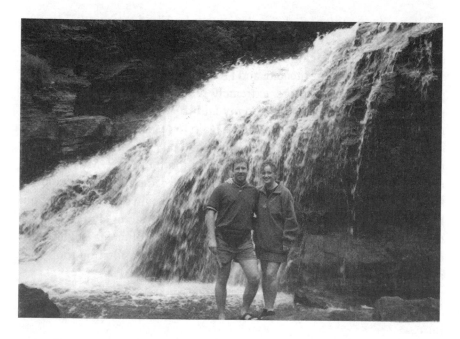

Anne and me in Canada in happier days

mouth, tongue and cheeks. I tried it. Nothing. My face felt extraordinarily heavy and my tongue seemed to be filling my mouth. Swallowing was still difficult but becoming slightly easier. I tried just opening and closing my mouth. It was no use. I couldn't get it to close all the way. My bottom jaw felt too heavy, and my bottom lip felt as if gravity was causing it to curl outward. I felt more saliva dribbling over my lip. I thought harder. What else did Kirk say he did? Wasn't there something about changing the pitch of the sounds? I tried grunting. Every sound was the same, low in pitch and completely monotone. I remembered his words. 'What use is an actor who can't talk?' I was genuinely moved when I saw him giving the television interview, but only when lying on that trolley did his words have real meaning. I immediately thought back to myself, and in my ignorance as to the possible consequences of my situation thought, 'What good is a teacher who can't speak? What good is a PE teacher who can't move?'

It was probably around this time I went cold as the seriousness of the situation sunk in. Forget about teaching, what if this was going to be the physical state I would be in for the rest of my life? I tried frantically to regain control of the muscles of my face, mouth and tongue. I was panicking too much to be grateful that at least I was still able to understand other people and think of the words that I wanted to use.

It was during this period of isolation that I realised, perhaps for the first time, that language is not a bolt-on extra to our daily routine that should be taken lightly. In the cold light of day, I believe that the work of speech therapists cannot be underestimated, and I remain amazed at the skills that they must possess. I was, therefore, extremely relieved when some time later a minor improvement with regard to my mouth and tongue happened very rapidly over a period of minutes. I tried again to open and close my jaw. My bottom jaw slammed into the top jaw, as I had no real control. I realised in the days that followed that this had caused a tooth to crack. My tongue, at that time, felt as if it had shrunk slightly, and I became aware that I could at last co-ordinate the right muscles in order to make myself be understood. My face and lips, however, remained very numb and, strangely, I have never really regained the normal feeling in my nose, which often feels numb with cold. The nurse, who had stayed with me, left the consultation room and returned with the doctor.

'How are you feeling now?' I was asked.

'A bit better,' was what I hoped could be understood, 'but my head hurts.'

My tongue felt thick and clumsy. The muscles in my neck and around my jaw seemed to be in spasm. It was still hard to swallow.

Again, the doctor shone a light into my eyes. I concentrated on keeping my head still as I was still shaking badly. I did not know then, but this medical assessment was something I would get used to over the following 36 hours and, due to one doctor's competence, led to me having a brain scan.

'Do you generally get many headaches?' I was asked.

'No.'

'Have you received any bumps on the head today?'

'No.'

The doctor sat on the stool and looked at me thoughtfully. I looked back and tried to appear dignified – despite the shaking, despite the sweat, despite my clothes and despite the vomit. The automatic BP monitor inflated tightly around my bicep again.

'Are you allergic to anything?'

'No,' I replied.

'Have you changed your eating habits recently?' was the next question.

'I did have quite a bit of chocolate over the Christmas holiday,' I answered.

'I'm not sure, without the aid of further tests, whether this is anything more than a migraine,' the doctor said. 'I think I'll discuss this with a colleague and we'll decide whether to keep you in for observation overnight. Shall I show your partner in while I'm gone?'

'Yes,' I replied.

Anne came into the consultation room with her sister. Anne had never learnt to drive and so she had telephoned her sister immediately after Paul had contacted her, a couple of hours earlier. She was obviously shocked to see me shaking uncontrollably and wired up to several machines.

Anne and I both had pastoral duties at school, which, combined with my involvement in extracurricular sports clubs, resulted in us not even meeting during break or lunch times. However, on the way home from work we would share accounts, mostly funny ones, of things that had happened in the day. One of my favourites includes when a young boy in her year group fainted during the two-minute silence on Armistice Day. This is not funny in itself, but afterwards he told the first aid staff on duty: 'I knew I was going to faint, but didn't think I was allowed to move, or speak, during the two-minute silence!'

The last time Anne had seen me I was in the gym and about to start the junior class of the martial arts club. Then, I was physically fit and confident. We were both ignorant of the difference a few hours would make. I am not sure of what exactly was said, but when she saw me in the hospital, Anne coped better than I was expecting her to – she is a worrier on matters to do with health. I was really glad to see her. To be truthful, it did not occur to me until some weeks later that if things had been slightly different we would never have seen each other again. Anne had the presence of mind to bring me my toiletry bag, which is permanently packed in a drawer in the bathroom for trips to the gym and short holiday breaks away. My speech was slow and laboured, and I had to focus carefully on what to say. Anne told me that my parents were on their way, and her sister went out into the corridor to wait for them to arrive. I was vomiting much less by the time Anne was with me, but my stomach muscles burned after hours of forced contractions. We talked about the previous few days. Anne reminded me that I had told her one morning, just a few days before, that a loud 'pop' from within my head, accompanied with a feeling that someone had thrown a dart into the back of my head, had woken me up during the night. An uncomfortable, though certainly not severe, neck pain and headache had remained. Unable to shake it off, I had simply taken a headache tablet and gone off to work as usual each day. Unknown to us then, this detail was to prove significant to my consultant some months later when he considered it in relation to a variety of health test results that all returned as negative.

My parents soon arrived and almost immediately the doctor who was looking after me confirmed that as a result of the second opinion she had sought, I would be kept in hospital overnight in order for some tests to be done the following day. To be honest, I was relieved at this course of action, as I don't believe I would have made it home. Two porters arrived, and I was transported, accompanied by my family party along dimly lit corridors, into a lift and up to the Acute Medical Unit (AMU: see Glossary) on the first floor. Once there, I was drifting in and out of consciousness and it was suggested to Anne and my parents that they leave almost immediately. There was nothing they could do and I'm glad that they went.

A strange thing happened to me in the AMU during the night. As I drifted in and out of what seemed like the twilight zone, several doctors came and shone their ophthalmoscopes into my eyes and my senses were stimulated by strange noises coming from different parts of the ward. One sound, close to me, caused me to wake and try to force my eyes open.

'No! Betty, stop!' I heard from somewhere.

'Indeed I won't,' came the reply from the face I now saw looking down on me from just a few centimetres away. The face was toothless, very cracked and surrounded by a halo of frizzy grey-white hair. It lowered towards me, lips puckered for a kiss. I remember trying to scream for help but nothing came out. I needed to create a distance between us and tried to force my head backwards, through the pillow supporting it. With just millimetres to go, a second head came into view. Thankfully, it was on the body of someone in a nurse's uniform.

'Come on now, Betty. You really must behave. I've told you before, leave the men alone. Let's get you back to your room and back to bed.'

And so Betty was led away, somewhat reluctantly.

I wondered what was happening to me as I fell back to sleep.

Sometime before the morning wake-up call at 7.30, part of me was aware that I was being moved to somewhere else in the hospital. I felt like I was an observer to this, watching from elsewhere. When I woke up I saw a smiling, white-haired man with unusually white dentures sitting on my bed. I am with Kirk Douglas, I thought, until I came to my senses and Frank introduced himself for the first time.

After I declined the offer of a sweet, and Frank had gone back to his bed, I was introduced to the morning routine in the hospital ward. The nursing duty team breezed in making jokes, talking to the patients and referring to them by name. Patients were encouraged to get out of their bed if they were able to do so, and sit in the armchair next to their bed. This was so that the bed could be made up and fitted with clean sheets. Those patients, like me, who were confined to bed were offered a wash and shave. I declined this service on that first occasion as I still felt like an observer to the events. Then came the distribution of medication. I was given a mix of pills, only caring that they contained painkillers for my headache. I felt like I had been hit at the base of my skull with a baseball bat. Next came the breakfast trolley with a choice of toast or cereal, accompanied with orange juice, tea or coffee. After a respite of about half an hour the doctors' rounds began.

A team surrounded my bed and the curtain was pulled around. I am not sure exactly how many there were, but I think six is a conservative estimate. The doctor in charge seemed concerned about my eyes, speech, reflexes and limb strength. I was amazed that despite the medical equipment every-where I was still asked to try to touch my nose with each index finger and then point to the doctor's finger. I didn't realise that the finger–nose test is used successfully in order to determine cerebellar brain damage or disease (the effects of stroke on different parts of the brain is examined in Chapter 9 'After a Stroke'). In addition, I had to try to follow the movements of the doctor's finger across my face with my eyes.

Following what I considered to be a fairly thorough examination, which involved trying to move, and co-ordinate various parts of my body, he told me he was going to arrange a *CT brain scan*. He said he was con-cerned about what he saw when looking into my eyes. This may have been due to symptoms relating to *nystagmus* or *ocular dysynergia*, although I was not told. He said that he hoped that the scan would be done that day, but could not promise anything. He informed me that if the brain scan showed nothing, I would have to have a *lumbar puncture*. And then as suddenly as they had arrived they were gone.

'Good doctor, him,' one of the male nurses said to me as he walked past my bed.

I did not answer. I realise now that I was in a state of shock. Brain scans. Lumbar punctures. I thought immediately of meningitis. I knew that a lumbar puncture was performed to check for meningitis. I thought back to a few years earlier when the school was directly affected by meningitis after the death of my colleague and friend, Lynne. This did not help ease my fears in the slightest.

The brain scan and confirmation of stroke

Later that first morning I was wheeled down to the X-ray department for my first test, referred to by the nurse as a CT scan. As we waited in the corri-

CT (computed tomography) brain scan is a computerised X-ray procedure that produces cross-sectional images of the brain. CT imaging, also known as 'CAT scanning' (computed axial tomography), is perhaps the doctor's method of choice for imaging trauma patients because: it has the ability to image a combination of soft tissue, bone, and blood vessels; it is fast, simple and enables a quick overview of possibly life-threatening pathology; due to the short scan times of 500 milliseconds to a few seconds, it can be used for all areas of the body, including those susceptible to patient movement and breathing; it enables the patient to receive rapid and dedicated surgical treatment; and the images are far more detailed than ordinary X-rays, and can reveal disease or abnormalities in tissue and bone.

Nystagmus refers to rapid involuntary movements of the eyes that may be from side to side, up and down, or rotary. Depending on the cause, these movements may be in both eyes or in just one eye.

Ocular dysynergia is a failure of either eye to move promptly, or smoothly. It is best tested by asking the patient to follow the slow movement of a visual target across the visual field.

Lumbar puncture (spinal tap) tests drain small samples of cerebral spinal fluid from the lower spine in order to test for associated problems. A needle is inserted between the vertebrae (backbones) in the lower back and into the space containing the spinal fluid and samples are collected.

dor, she told me that CT images of the head are helpful in detecting tumours, blood clots and blood vessel defects, enlarged ventricles, and other abnormalities, such as those of the nerves or muscles of the eye.

The procedure was completely painless, relatively brief and I was relieved that nothing was stuck into me. The technologist positioned me on the specialised CT table. The area of medical interest, my head, was placed in a special holder that extended around my head and neck. Soft straps were used to help position and immobilise my head and ensure that a precise scan was possible. I was then slid inside the CT gantry opening, which looked like a big keyhole. Once I was comfortably and correctly positioned, I was encouraged to lie still and relax. The technologist left me (the CT technologist controls the CT examination from a workstation console in the next room) and I shut my eyes. I heard some whirring as the scanner rotated around me and acquired the necessary data. Later that day, the results would be processed and eventually passed on to the doctors who requested the scan. Soon I was back on the ward and back in my bed.

Before long, I pressed the alarm next to my bed and was pleased that the sister in charge came to me.

'Please don't let any children from my school in to visit, should they show up,' I said. Earlier, as I was having the CT scan, I had suddenly remembered one of my colleagues telling me that when she came round from having an operation for gall stones, she had woken to find one of her 13-year-old pupils sitting in the chair next to the bed smiling at her.

'Hello, Miss,' the pupil had said. 'My father has just dropped me off. He'll be back in two hours to pick me up.' Even feeling as ill as I did at that moment, I could not think of a worse scenario than that one!

Later that morning I had several samples of blood taken. The *phlebotomist* told me that as it was a Friday I would not get the results of any of the blood tests until the following Monday. She confirmed that I had 'good veins' and that my blood would be tested for a variety of things. Again, as with the CT scan, it would be some days before the results would come back to me. As the phlebotomist left with my blood, Ken asked how I was bearing up.

'I don't know,' I replied. 'I don't know why I am here, but I feel so ill I'm just glad I am!'

Ken had been admitted with chest pains. He had suffered a heart attack several months earlier and was pleased to have been kept in hospital as it meant that he would see his specialist well in advance of his scheduled outpatient appointment.

As Ken and I were talking, a different team of doctors to that which I had seen earlier, now led by a consultant *endocrinologist*, Dr Evans, was with me at my bed. The curtain around my bed was pulled closed by Dr Evans, as if it would provide soundproofing and privacy, and I was examined again. I was asked a series of questions relating to my health and lifestyle, which were very straightforward and I was consequently able to answer.

No, I did not smoke.

No, I did not drink much alcohol.

Yes, I thought I was generally in good health. No, there was no family history of illness.

No, I was not allergic to anything that I was aware of. No, I was not unusually thirsty.

No, I was not urinating more regularly than usual.

Eventually, Dr Evans gave me the opportunity to ask him anything.

'So I'll be kept in?' was the best I could manage. My speech was still improving and I was pleased to be able to speak in sentences.

'Yes, but we'll get your results as soon as we possibly can,' he replied.

Phlebotomists draw blood from patients or blood donors for medical testing.

Endocrinologists diagnose and treat conditions of the endocrine system – a system of glands, including the thyroid, parathyroid, pancreas, ovaries, testes, adrenal, pituitary and hypothalamus glands. Glands are organs that make hormones (see Glossary), which in turn help to control reproduction, metabolism (food burning and waste elimination), and growth and development. Conditions treated by endocrinologists include: diabetes, thyroid diseases, metabolic problems, hormonal imbalances, menopause, osteoporosis, hypertension, cholesterol (lipid) disorders, infertility, shortness (short stature), and cancers of the glands.

I became slightly embarrassed, still thinking that all this fuss was to confirm that I'd had a migraine, probably caused by eating too much chocolate at Christmas!

It was afternoon when Anne and my parents arrived. I tried to tell them the tale of Betty, introduced them to Ken and recounted the morning's activities. Anne had somehow found herself going to work that first morning, but ended up getting upset when our colleagues asked how I was.

Anne, and my parents, were pleased that the CT had been done but they seemed more concerned about the results than me. I was simply trying to cope with the immediate and constant discomfort I was in. The back of my head hurt like I had been hit with a metal bar. Actually, hit very hard with a metal bar. Fortunately, before too long I was allowed more painkillers and given some extra, different ones, for good measure. The pain left me slightly, and so I was forced to deal only with the dizziness. As I lay in my bed I felt like I was on a boat in the worst swell in the worst storm. To try to combat the feeling, I gripped the sheets so hard my knuckles were white. I had visions of falling off the bed and was unable to sit upright. Unfortunately, this feeling, known as *truncal ataxia*, was overpowering. It was with me very strongly throughout my time in hospital, and actually kept returning intermittently for some months.

Anne was understandably sympathetic as to how I felt; however, she was equally concerned that I was still in very sweaty, vomit-stained training clothes and pointed out that she had brought some shorts and a clean T-shirt for me to wear. As far as I was concerned it would have to wait. I was unwashed and certainly unclean, but I couldn't support my head unaided and just wanted to lie still. So, I just lay there while Anne and my parents sat round me. Again, I drifted in and out of consciousness. The afternoon went by and soon it was the end of visiting time. I was pleased that they had been there, but was also pleased to become a fairly anonymous patient in Ward

12 when they left. It was Friday night but I was pleased to be able to go to sleep early.

It was the following morning that I was woken by a nurse I recognised from the ward, who was accompanied by a doctor I had previously seen with Dr Evans. It was then that I was told I had suffered an *ischaemic stroke* caused by a blood clot. I wasn't given any indication as to whether the stroke was a minor one or a major one, but I learnt later that minor strokes, caused by a blockage rather than a bleed, often do not show up on a CT scan. In addition, some reports state that less than 50 per cent of ischemic strokes are evident on CT scans within the first 24 hours.

Truncal ataxia is an inability to maintain an upright position, and is a feature of midline cerebellar disease.

Ischaemic stroke is a stroke caused by a blockage of an artery or blood vessel, which interrupts blood flow to the brain. This is the most common category (by cause) of stroke and is also called a cerebral infarction.

The doctor explained, 'As it's the weekend not much will be happening for a couple of days. You need to stay quite still, and remain in bed. The staff will look after you. There will be more tests next week and you'll meet with the physiotherapist, occupational therapist, and the stroke specialist nurse. Here are some leaflets and literature about strokes for you and your family to look at. I'll leave them in your bedside drawer.'

'Do you want us to tell your partner and parents the results of the scan when they come in?' the nurse asked. I was grateful for the offer, but it was something I had to do myself. Somehow!

'No thanks, I'll tell them when they turn up. Anne will be less worried if I am able to tell her myself,' I said, before I started recalling all the people I knew who had had a stroke.

As I lay on the hospital bed, it was as if time had stood still. I was worried that as a person I had regressed, becoming physically and consciously incompetent, as opposed to the level of competence I had enjoyed all of my life. I was not concerned, at this stage, about complex skills, just those competences I had taken for granted. I thought of the simple things like rising from a chair, walking, and climbing a staircase. I thought hard about when my ability to speak and swallow had been lost in a second just a matter of hours before.

Ken asked me if there was any news as to why I was in hospital. I realised that I had been completely absorbed in my thoughts for some time.

'Yes, I've had a stroke.'

It was the first time I had said the words. I was thankful that my speech was better than it had been but wished that I didn't have to say those words. I was still relieved that I was able to speak at all, so it took some of the pain out of admitting that I had finally become vulnerable. Even though we had just met, Ken's face was one of shock. Shock was a reaction I had to get used to over the next few weeks. The many phone calls, cards and messages from friends and relatives all started with a statement of absolute shock. In truth saying the words meant nothing to me. This was despite the fact that I was well educated, despite seeing Kirk Douglas on the television, despite the fact I had had an indirect association with stroke through my family since a young boy, despite the fact that I even made reference to strokes as part of a physiology course I taught at school. Despite all this, I still did not really understand anything about stroke or what had happened to me.

I was very keen not to still be in the same clothes when Anne arrived the next day. I would have been wearing them for the third day running. I found myself wanting to be presentable and create a good impression when I told her the news. I suppose I thought that it might, in some way, soften the blow. Despite the offer of a bed bath from the nurses, I wanted some privacy, which perhaps further illustrated my unexpected and sudden vulnerability. A male nurse from the ward was called to take me to the shower room. He helped me out of bed and onto the commode. He took his time, talked to me constantly and was patient as I tried to reply.

As I sat on the commode in the shower room he helped to undress me and we established that he had gone to school at one of my school's close sporting rivals and where one of my best friends was Head of Physical Education. Despite the fact I had to be helped to shower, wash and dry I felt comfortable with him. It is amazing how difficult standing up is, when you have to think about it. I told him that I would be able to handle the shower's handset and promptly lost control, soaking him and pinning him against the wall with the water jet. It was a truly absurd sight. So, with me dressed in my clean shorts and T-shirt, the nurse, with his uniform dripping wet, wheeled me towards the door. I will remember the next moment as long as I live. For some reason I shut my eyes as the mirror approached, not wanting to look at myself. I could not bear to see what might be looking back at me. This was a reaction I still cannot fully explain. I knew that I had not been disfigured in any way, but I was not ready to see the new me, without my disguise. I remember thinking, I bet my uncles and Kirk Douglas coped better than this.

Going to the shower that morning, washing, dressing and getting back to bed was one of the most physically demanding tasks I have ever done.

Some accepted risk factors for stroke – do any of these apply to you?

- High blood pressure
- Contributory factors to high blood pressure (smoking, high alcohol consumption, stress, physical inactivity)
- Narrow arteries
- Contributory factors to narrow arteries (poor diet, diabetes, physical inactivity)
- Heart disease
- Previous stroke or transient ischaemic attack (TIA)
- Age (older people are generally at greater risk)
- Ethnicity (stroke is common throughout the world, but people of Asian and Afro-Caribbean origin are at higher risk)
- Genetics (people with a family history of stroke are more vulnerable)
- Oral contraceptives
- History of migraine (in women)

Just 48 hours earlier I would have been capable of completing activity that required physical strength, power, balance, agility, co-ordination and dexterity. I reiterate this only to illustrate the fact that a significant change had occurred to me. Surprisingly, I was still not dwelling on the fact that I could not do these things. I was now dwelling on having to tell Anne that I had had a stroke. What would she think of me? I was no longer the person she had started to share her life with. Things were relatively comfortable for us. We worked together, spent most evenings and weekends together and were able to do what we wanted to when we wanted to do it. Had all that stopped?

Anne arrived with my father a couple of hours later, around midday. They sat down and Anne asked how I was.

I took a deep breath and managed to say, for the second time in my life, 'I've had a stroke.' I added, 'There are some leaflets there if you want to see, but I can't face looking at them.'

The colour on my father's face drained away. I don't think he has spent a day in hospital in life. He had several visits for broken bones playing football, for a tetanus jab after being kicked by a horse (an animal lover, my father maintains that it was his fault not the horse's) and even for stitches as a result of a game of squash, but what he didn't do was illness.

'I'll phone your mother,' he said, and before I could stop him left the ward. Anne reached over to me and hugged me. We shared a moment that I will never forget, and I somehow felt better despite the fact that once again the painkillers were wearing off.

'What does it mean?' Anne asked.

'I don't know,' I said.

'Are there more tests?'

'I think so, Monday maybe.'

'What type of stroke?'

'I don't know. A specialist stroke nurse will be coming to see me.'

'Why didn't they tell us?'

'That was my idea, I thought it would be better coming from me. I knew you'd be brave in front of me and thought that that way you wouldn't feel as bad.'

'I'm a bit scared,' Anne said.

'Don't be, I'm scared enough for both of us!' There, I said it. I had admitted I was scared by something. I added, 'Anyway, it could have been worse. It could have happened at the start of a holiday, not at the start of a teaching term!'

My father came back in and told us that my mother was on her way. I didn't want him to ring her, as she would now be driving in to see me, distracted and probably distressed. However, on reflection I know and accept that my father had to tell her immediately as it was his way of confronting the situation. He probably also wanted to give Anne and me a moment together. I had no more answers or information to give them. So, strange as it was, we didn't really talk about the stroke until my mother arrived. After the hugging and kissing, which I noticed would have been exactly the same reaction to good news, my mother asked the same questions that Anne had. As I answered them again, a voice in my head was telling me over and over again: 'Today is the first day of the rest of your life.' I felt strangely peaceful despite the confusion.

We eventually talked of visitors and telling other people. I had decided while I was waiting for them all to arrive that I did not want any visitors while I was in hospital. This was not because I didn't want people to see me, in the same way that I could not look at myself in the mirror. Simply, I didn't know what had really happened, why it had happened, how I felt, what risk I was in, or what the future would now hold. The exceptions, I decided, were to be Paul and Mark. I was certainly in a better condition than when they had seen me loaded into the ambulance, and I thought that they needed to know I was surviving (Mark especially!). Anyone else could wait until I got home, however long it would take. As it turned out, Mark had to spend most of the next three days at the same hospital with his very ill grandfather, so he called to see me several times. Mark's grandfather had been admitted to the AMU ward where I had spent half the first night. Unfortunately, he died a few days later.

The next few days in hospital were understandably uneventful. After a reasonable night's sleep, occasionally interrupted by the headache and need for more painkillers, I would wake up at 7.30 when I was given a high dose of aspirin and painkillers. Ken and I would update each other as to how we felt and how we slept. Frank, looking a picture of health, would wander over and update us as to how he slept and felt. Ken would repeat to Frank what he had told me, and then it would be my turn. After everyone else had used the bathroom I would be put on the commode by the male nurse and wheeled over to it. Every day I would try to control the shower

Hospital visiting – tips for visitors to the Stroke Ward

- Do tell the medical staff of all medical conditions the patient has.
- Don't expect doctors to make accurate predictions concerning recovery early on.
- Don't feel the need to talk to the patient all of the time.
- If the patient has verbal communication difficulties, use touch and facial expressions as you talk and remember that as much as 70 per cent communication is non-verbal.
- A simple telephone message to the ward at the start of each day can be uplifting to the patient.
- Do talk to the nursing staff about ward routines, care and medication – possibly ask if you can help.
- Try to keep a sense of humour.
- When not visiting, talk to family and friends and do try to do something uplifting for yourself.

and every day we would both end up soaking wet. And every day I managed to avoid looking in the mirror.

I went into hospital with a beard on my chin. After a few days I needed a shave to freshen up. It was too difficult to shave both the right and left sides of my face with my right hand, and I had even less success with my left hand. A combination of not being able to co-ordinate the muscles to shave around the beard and not wanting to look in the mirror meant that one day I emerged from the bathroom clean shaven. I was still plagued with a violent headache, dizziness and feeling sick, despite the medication and variety of painkillers. On the positive side, I didn't lose my appetite and ate well throughout the day.

Some time over the course of these days and for the following weeks, my relationship with my mother regressed some 35 years. She became most interested, almost to the point of obsession, with whether I had had a 'bowel movement', as the medical team liked to call it. This is not a term I tended to use much myself! When questioned, I realised that I had not had a 'bowel movement' since being admitted to hospital, and was indeed constipated.

Around half of all people have bowel problems at some time in their lives. The digestive system is sensitive to changes in lifestyle, so you should not be surprised when, for whatever reason, things start to move more slowly than usual. I remembered, a few years earlier, when a young boy was finding the transition from the junior school to high school traumatic. He had not had a bowel movement for weeks and was given laxatives by his parents, the result being that his system resumed normal progress when I was teaching him gymnastics!

I think that the most important thing about constipation is probably not to worry. However, I was worried. I was genuinely worried that if I continued to be constipated the strain of my system 'kick starting' itself might induce another stroke.

As I did not remember the first time I had been potty trained, this sudden interest from my mother took some getting used to, especially as she seemed fairly indiscreet in her enquiries and the whole ward and their visitors became aware of my situation. I had never needed a laxative before and I became interested as to what was available. To my amazement I learned that there are several different types of oral laxatives and they work in different ways. I seemed to find most talk of laxatives and 'bowel movements' hilarious, which I was able to put down to a side-effect of the stroke. Later, we were told that it would be likely that I would start laughing or crying uncontrollably or uncharacteristically as a result of the stroke. On reflection, the truth is I always found this subject humorous, but now had an excuse for my schoolboy mentality. The description 'bulk-formers' conjured up various graphic images in my mind, which was at that time being stimulated far less than usual. Apparently, bulk-forming laxatives are also used to treat diarrhoea. I can't imagine a visit to the doctor to sort out a diarrhoea problem and ending up with a laxative prescription!

I also found the terms 'lubricants' and 'stimulants' amusing. I was given a sickly sweet laxative called lactulose (see Glossary) with my breakfast and with my evening meal. Lactulose falls under the category of a hyperosmotic laxative and is available only with a doctor's prescription. Lactulose is a special sugar-like laxative used for rapid emptying of the lower intestine and bowel. It encourages bowel movements by drawing water into the bowel from surrounding body tissues, providing a soft stool mass and increased bowel action. However, it produces results slowly and is often used for long-term treatment of chronic constipation.

As the days went by, encouraged by my mother's interest, I began to think I should have been prescribed what are medically termed 'stool softeners' or emollients. These are said not to cause a bowel movement but instead allow the patient to have a bowel movement without straining. I was fortunate really – a quarter of stroke survivors become incontinent of faeces for some time as a result of constipation or damage to the part of the brain controlling bowel movements.

As it turned out, hospital was not the place for me to have a successful 'bowel movement' and the medication presented to me when I was discharged several days later included a large bottle of lactulose, which I continued to take diligently. I am only too pleased that my mother was visiting me at home when my digestive system started working again, as it saved me from having to make a special telephone call to her. As I sat, I wondered for a moment whether Kirk Douglas had had the same problems.

Religion finds me!

'I do benefits for all religions – I'd hate to blow the hereafter on a technicality.'

Bob Hope

While in hospital, and in between worrying about everything else, I was forced to consider my religious beliefs. My religious denomination, though sometimes a thoroughly confusing and frustrating thing to care about, is perfectly clear. I was baptised as one of the billion Catholics in the world and brought up as a Catholic. It has been a source of family amusement over the years that my pet budgie, Sooty, died during the night of 28 September 1978. This was the same night as Pope John Paul I died, leaving my father in a quandary regarding his duty – specifically, who he should tell me about first! I don't think it really mattered, as the loss of a friendly budgie was always going to be more disappointing to a 12-year-old boy.

I eventually ended up teaching in a Catholic school, which I do believe can have unique features and ethos. In order for Catholic schools to promote themselves and be sustained in our society, evidence of community spirit cannot be an option. It should visibly exist, being welcomed and promoted by those people interacting with each other. At times, this requires a degree of faith. Throughout my life, I have witnessed the power of faith in people around me, both young and old. It is not easy to have faith, and this itself requires a 'leap of faith'. Faith, however, is universal among religions, with each being an arbitrary attempt to comprehend all that is greater than mankind. I do not believe in everything that man says about God, but I do believe in God and that life has a meaning. However, I feel that attending church is at times little more than candlelight monotony. While many churchgoers actively strive to make their community a better place, I have found over the years that many of the people who contribute to the church as an institution are certainly not for me. Catholic, by definition, is a very inclusive word and yet the Catholic Church as an institution is divided on how inclusive it should be in today's global society. There is a presumption from many individuals, including ordained and lay members, that the advice and opinions they offer should be accepted on their terms and without condition. Anne was with me in hospital during one such occasion. My lunch had just arrived and I was just lifting my cutlery off the tray when a tall nun walked in and invited herself to sit with us. I replaced my cutlery out of politeness. She introduced herself as a sister and a 'friend of the hospital'. She had selected me for a visit based on my admission profile, which stated my religion as well as name, address, date of birth and other details. She obviously meant well but her visit was mistimed, naïve and, to be honest, inappropriate. I was still very weak, emotionally fragile, confused as to what was happening to me and anxious about what the future had in store. Anne was exhausted and hadn't slept properly for four or five days. In her Irish accent, and speaking without a breath, she talked at us for close to 15 minutes.

'Hello to you. I'll spend some time with you, now. I visit this hospital from Newport where the convent is. Your name is McCann? Would your father be Brian? If it is, he knows my sister.'

At this point I was confused as to whether she had a sister, or whether she was referring to the other nuns in the convent. I didn't have time to ponder on this for long, as she continued, 'Yes. I like this hospital. It's a good hospital. Very new! Very clean! Well, whatever is the matter with you?'

'I've had a stroke.' I said it for just the third time.

'A stroke. Sure, you're very young! Nice staff here. The Canon visits here too. Do you know the Canon? He loves the sick, loves them! He'll be in later in the week. I'll leave him a note to come and see you. You should have the Last Sacrament! It's not called the Last Rites or the Sacrament of the Dying any more. It's called the Sacrament of the Sick. It's much better. It offers great healing. Great healing!'

I realise that a religion that does not help people to meet the tragedies and trials of life would be of no use, and all religions pay attention to human suffering. However, to me the Sacrament of the Sick was still the Last Rites given to those about to die, and I did not want it. I did not have a problem with my beliefs, just a problem accepting my newly established vulnerability. All world religions are on common ground in including suffering in their ideology, and I wondered briefly whether serious illness was just God's way of recruiting more charity workers, as most of the ones I had met had been affected by one form of illness or other, directly or indirectly.

She continued, 'There was a young man on the floor below us here. Dying. Dying he was. Of cancer! He hadn't eaten for days. Weak as a kitten! He received the Sacrament of the Sick. The oil rubbed on the head has healing qualities. The very next morning he was only sitting in bed eating Weetabix! Yes, Weetabix!'

At this point, despite the stroke, we somehow found the strength not to laugh out loud. Faith is a strong concept and I address the issue of prayer as a means of support in Chapter 10 'A Toolkit for Recovery and Prevention'. I have absolutely no doubt that the nun's story is based on some truth that miracles have happened and do happen, but her visit to me seemed most surreal – even now, 18 months later.

She continued without a pause, 'One poor lady was in here with her three sons. The Cancer! She lost all of them. Be grateful you don't have that!'

With this she left as suddenly as she had arrived. I turned to Anne and mumbled, 'I wonder if he can play the piano now as well!'

The time to laugh was now with us, and Anne and I were still laughing when my mother arrived half an hour later. It may have been due, in part, to the fact that Anne started to mimic the nun, and continued to remain 'in character' for quite some time! Even at this time I was able to relax, see the funny side of things and enjoy moments of spontaneous humour. This was a great help to me, psychologically speaking. It probably even induced some physiological responses to ease the pain. Some studies have demonstrated that laughter can significantly lower stress hormones and stimulate the body's natural antibodies (e.g. Berk 1989).

The Canon did, in fact, arrive some days later. Fortunately, I saw him coming through the glass window at the nurses' desk, which was just outside the doors into the ward. The school I worked in was based in his parish, and as a result he was often a visitor to the school. In fact, he was chairman of the school's governing body when I was interviewed for my first job at the school just after I qualified as a teacher in 1989.

As much as I liked him, I did not want to see him. I had made a decision regarding visitors and even my closest friends were not visiting me. Ken and I were in mid-conversation as he approached the ward. I suddenly shut my eyes and pretended to fall asleep. It was not uncommon for me to fall asleep at that time, and so Ken just picked up his paper and began to read. I was not in the mood for another religious visit and I still did not want to receive the Sacrament of the Sick. Unfortunately, this did not deter the Canon who tried to wake me up. To an observer, things would have looked a bit odd. Me, a 37-year-old man acting like a mischievous seven-year-old by suddenly pretending to fall asleep. Nevertheless, he was persistent. As he shook my arm I remembered the words of the nun, 'He loves the sick!' I knew then he would not be going away.

I heard Ken saying, 'Excuse me, he's just fallen asleep, probably best to leave him.' The Canon was having none of it and he started to tap my arm as well. I decided to get it over with, and put on a show of waking up from a deep sleep that a pantomime actor would have been proud of.

Like the nun before him, the Canon told me several stories of critically ill, dying people and added some about particularly good funerals for good measure. He was obviously very disappointed when I again declined to receive the Sacrament of the Sick. Eventually he left, promising to call back in to see me on his next scheduled visit.

As I lay there after he had gone, I had to accept that I had been stimulated into thinking about one thing I had tried to push out of my mind – death.

I am unlike many people in that thinking of death often makes me laugh. This is because it inevitably leads to thinking of funerals, which reminds me of Anne's father. Her father, Ed, died suddenly in 2002, and he is greatly missed by all who knew him. However, for the last few years of his life she described him as a 'professional funeral groupie'. He loved a good funeral. The first time I met him he had just been to what he described as an exceptionally enjoyable funeral. He told me, 'Kath [Anne's sister] was crying. The wife was crying. The daughter was crying. I thoroughly enjoyed it!' Apparently, there was a blues band playing and Ed liked music.

One of his favourite stories was concerning a funeral (he actually missed it, much to his disappointment!) of a man in the village where he lived. 'Only problem was,' he told me, 'he was about 20 stone! The bearers had to get him downstairs from his bedroom to the living room for the wake. Unfortunately, there was a right angle on the stairs and it was difficult to manoeuvre him round the bend. It was too much for one of the men as they were all getting on a bit and he dropped him, causing the body to emit some wind. "That's it," the bearer said, "if he can fart he can walk!" So, despite my own situation, thinking of Ed and his stories lifted my spirits tremendously when I was in hospital, and I missed the fact that he was not around to visit me.

As I lay dwelling on thoughts of death and funerals, as brought on by my unsolicited visitors, I formulated the premise on which I was determined to base my recovery. Whatever the tests showed, and whatever the doctors told me, I was glad that I was alive and not dead. With this at the forefront of my mind I would cope. I can't say with any honesty that I would have continued to feel the same if my stroke had rendered me paralysed, as I also realised that I was more scared of being incapacitated than of dying. On this point I have heard it said that stroke is the biggest fear among doctors, as they know only too well that paralysis is one of the likely consequences of stroke. There is even a 2005 health advertising campaign designed to encourage individuals to have a cholesterol check which starts with the statement, 'You can live with your diabetes: but could you live with a STROKE?'

As time went by on the ward, I could not concentrate on anything and was unable to enjoy the ward's communal television. I could not see properly and was too dizzy and unable to focus in order to read. Yet time did not seem to go slowly. I lay thinking or lay sleeping for most of the time. Strangely, I was neither very happy nor very sad. Occasionally, I broke off from my thoughts by putting on my bedside radio. I enjoyed one item in particular, which was focusing on a financial journalist and his new website which offered free money-saving advice. I resolved then to sort out my financial affairs when I was released from hospital.

The next few days were taken up with more tests and the inevitable worry of '…what if the results come back positive?' mixed with further worry and uncertainty along the lines of '...if the results are negative, why did it happen?' Although at that time I didn't really want to know more about what a stroke actually was, I needed to know what had caused my stroke. I had resigned myself to the adjustments that would have to be made to my life, and the possibility of not being able to participate in physical activity as I had before. The ease with which I accepted all this surprised me and demonstrated that maybe the experience was having a profound effect on me even then. I didn't know these things for certain, I was just preparing myself for what was fairly obviously the case. I also had serious doubts about returning to my teaching job.

I thought about holidays. Anne and I had travelled around Canada or Alaska every summer for the previous five years. We had participated in white-water rafting, canoeing, walking and whale watching. Would I be able to fly? Would I be able to cope with the pace of such holidays? If not able to work, would I be able to afford such holidays? Again, I accepted that I might not be able to do these things any more with surprising ease. The pace of my lifestyle had changed literally overnight, and as a consequence so had my priorities for happiness and fulfilment.

> 'There are two ways to live your life. One is as though nothing is a miracle. The other is as though everything is a miracle.'
>
> *Albert Einstein*

Some tests to establish the cause

The next time I left the ward was when I was wheeled out for a series of tests designed to establish why I had a stroke as the result of a blood clot. As I said in the Introduction, the concept of stroke can get complicated. Stroke is a term that relates to brain damage but it also related to the cause, the signs and the symptoms. In terms of my stroke, where had the clot come from? Why had it formed? Could it happen again? I was, of course, only too pleased for any tests to be conducted.

The first test took approximately 20 minutes and was a painless *carotid artery ultrasound scan*. This is a common scan for stroke patients because a stroke most often occurs when the carotid arteries become blocked and the brain does not get enough oxygen – known as *atherosclerosis*. Despite my nerves at the possible outcome, I found this test interesting as I could hear the sound of the blood flow and see the images displayed on the monitor. I was told immediately that all was well, which was a relief because I had been extremely worried at the thought of surgery if the readings were positive. Surgery, I had been warned, would probably have been in the form of a

Carotid artery ultrasound scan is also known as a carotid duplex ultrasound. It assesses blood flow in the carotid arteries, which lead to the brain, and detects any narrowing (as caused by plaque) or blockages (such as blood clots). After a water-soluble gel is applied to the skin of the neck, a device called a transducer, which directs high-frequency sound waves (ultrasound) into the carotid arteries, is rubbed lightly over the neck. Soundwaves, at frequencies that correspond to the velocity of blood flow, are reflected back to the machine and converted into audible sounds and graphic recordings.

Atherosclerosis is a narrowing of arteries due to the build up of plaques. This is the most common cause of both heart attack (coronary arteries) and stroke (typically, carotid and vertebral arteries; however, people of African and Asian descent often have trouble with the arteries within the skull). It is one of several risk factors for individuals who suffer both heart attack and stroke.

Carotid endarterectomy is a one- to three-hour surgical procedure to remove fatty plaque from neck arteries. It has a 40-year track record and over this period has become used increasingly as a stroke prevention measure. While the patient is under anaesthesia, surgeons make an incision in the neck, at the location of the blockage. A tube is inserted above and below the blockage to reroute blood flow. Surgeons can then open up the carotid artery and remove the plaque. Once the artery is stitched closed, the tube is removed.

carotid endarterectomy. While this is a treatment that has been proven safe and effective in providing long-term benefits to patients, I really didn't want it.

The second test I had was another completely painless test, an *echocardiogram*. For this, I was wheeled to a different part of the hospital. A trained sonographer usually performs the test, the results of which are then interpreted by a doctor. In my case, a doctor, one of the consultant's team, actually conducted the test. An echocardiogram works well for most patients and allows the doctor to see the heart beating and to visualise many of the structures of the heart.

An abnormal echocardiogram may indicate *atrial fibrillation*; *cardiomyopathy*; *congenital heart disease*; fluid in the sac around the heart; heart valve disease; or any other heart abnormalities. Again, I was relieved that my test results were clear.

Following the echocardiogram, I was pushed to the X-ray department for chest X-rays, another painless procedure. While the chest X-ray would also highlight any lung problems, in my case the focus was on the heart. Once again, all was clear.

Days earlier, during one of his first examinations, the consultant endocrinologist, Dr Evans, had told me he wanted to conduct further blood

Echocardiogram uses soundwaves to create a moving picture of the heart and is the quickest, safest test available to give information about the heart. The picture is much more detailed than an X-ray image and involves no exposure to radiation. It is good for monitoring the heart after a heart attack and can diagnose some types of heart disease; find tumours; and find blood clots in the upper chambers of the heart. The patient lies on the left side of the body on a padded table and a water soluble gel is applied to the skin around the heart. A transducer, transmitting high-frequency soundwaves, is then placed on the ribs near the breast bone and directed towards the heart. These impulses are then converted into moving pictures of the heart. Occasionally, because of the lungs, ribs or body tissue the soundwaves and echoes may be prevented from providing a clear picture of heart function. In such cases a small amount of a dye through an intravenous drip may be administered to improve the image of the inside of the heart. Very rarely, more invasive testing using special echocardiography probes may be necessary. For such an event a *transoesophageal echocardiogram* (TEE) is used. This involves the back of the throat being anaesthetised and a scope being inserted down the throat. On the end of the scope is an ultrasonic device that an experienced technician will guide down to the lower part of the oesophagus, where it is used to obtain a more clear two-dimensional echocardiogram of the heart.

Atrial fibrillation is a heartbeat irregularity causing blood clots to form in the heart itself.

Cardiomyopathy is a disease of the heart muscle that causes it to lose its pumping strength. There can be many causes.

Congenital heart disease is a heart defect or condition present at birth.

tests to determine whether I was diabetic, which may have been a contributory factor to the stroke.

Diabetes was something I knew a little about, and I had often doubted whether or not I would be able to cope with an illness like diabetes. I have worked, through sport, quite extensively with children and adults with diabetes who do not seem to have let it affect them in any way, and I was also impressed with the positive attitude of a cousin who found out she was diabetic at 21 years old. Dr Evans told me that the results of the *blood sugar test* taken when I was first admitted to hospital showed *hyperglycaemia*. This, he explained, could have been a result of the physiological stress my body was under during the stroke, or it could be a sign of diabetes. A second blood sample, taken days later, showed that my blood sugar levels were normal. However, he thought it sensible to have a third test for reliability purposes and arranged for me to have it.

Blood sugar tests are done primarily to diagnose and evaluate a person with diabetes mellitus. The most common is the oral glucose tolerance test (OGTT). This involves an overnight fast; a blood sample after the fast; drinking a solution containing a prescribed amount of glucose; a two-hour wait; and a second blood sample.

Hyperglycaemia is abnormally high levels of glucose in the blood.

From studying physiology at university, I was aware of some basic facts relating to diabetes and I include them here, as some studies suggest that there is a strong link between diabetes and ischaemic stroke. Most dietary carbohydrate eventually ends up as glucose (see Glossary) in the blood, and the body uses glucose to supply the energy it needs to function. Insulin (see Glossary) is constantly made by the pancreas, making it easy for glucose to move from the blood into the cells of the body. When insulin is active, blood glucose levels fall and sugar from body tissues is stored in the form of glycogen. When glycogen is active, blood glucose levels rise. After a meal, blood glucose levels rise sharply. The pancreas then responds by releasing enough insulin to take care of all the newly added sugar found in the body. The insulin moves the sugar out of the blood and into the cells. It is then that the blood sugar starts to level off and fall. Any excess glucose is converted to *triglycerides* for energy storage by the liver and skeletal muscles. However, some cells, for example the brain and red blood cells, are almost totally dependent on blood glucose as a source of energy. The brain, in fact, requires that glucose concentrations in the blood remain within a certain range in order to function normally. As a result, a person with diabetes (specifically, type I) may have an insulin reaction in an instant, seeming perfectly normal one second and becoming unconscious the next. The early warning signs of this type of reaction are hunger, dizziness, sweating, confusion, palpitation, and numbness or tingling of the lips. If left untreated, the insulin-dependent diabetic may also experience double vision, trembling and disorientation, may perform strange actions, and may eventually lose consciousness.

Triglycerides are types of fat and are similar to cholesterol in that they too are found naturally in the blood. They are essential to the body and are used to provide energy. However, raised levels can cause health problems. Simply speaking, triglyceride levels can increase, or be elevated, as a result of too much sugar and alcohol in the diet.

I was obviously not aware of this at the time, but I have since come to learn of one stroke survivor who was actually in hospital for a diabetes test when he suffered a cerebellar stroke. Anyway, having exhibited many of the symptoms of diabetes in the hours surrounding the stroke I was comfortable with the fact that this needed to be either confirmed or discounted. Like the other tests, and to my relief, this too came back as normal.

Meeting the stroke nurse

I had been in hospital for five days when the specialist stroke nurse, Gill, came to see me. My parents and Anne were with me at the time. Gill informed us that the CT scan illustrated that I had suffered my stroke as a result of a blood clot that restricted the blood flow to the part of the brain called the cerebellum. I learned that this detail set me apart from many other stroke sufferers. Cerebellar stroke survivors are actually in the minority, as most strokes are cerebral. The cerebellum, accounting for 10 per cent of the brain's weight, is at the base of the brain (this is expanded on in more detail in Chapter 7 'The Brain and Its Blood Supply'). Strokes involving the cerebellum often involve the brainstem, and are sometimes classified by some as a brainstem stroke. This is because the arteries supplying the cerebellum also supply the medulla and brainstem. Some cerebellar stroke victims, particularly if they have, or develop, a chest infection, have been known to be unable to breathe unaided and needed a tracheotomy and, both brainstem and cerebellar strokes, have proven fatal.

The cerebellum contains more neurones in it than the rest of the brain. It may be that the cerebellum is involved with cognitive understanding, emotion and aspects of memory. However, it is mainly considered to be responsible for co-ordination, fine motor control (delicate or skilled voluntary movement), posture, balance and gait. The cerebellum operates automatically, without intruding into consciousness, and is involved in a feedback loop as motor impulses from the cerebrum are organised and transmitted to muscles. As the muscle tissue responds, its sensory nerve cells return information to the cerebellum.

Therefore, throughout periods of muscular activity, the cerebellum adjusts speed, force, and other factors involved in movement. With such an important role, the cerebellum accounts for over half the brain's population of neurones and receives impulses from all aspects of the central nervous system. It has been described as acting more like a brake than a motor, by preventing limbs from flailing about out of control. The overall effect of the continuous feedback loop is a smooth, balanced muscular activity. If the cerebellum is injured, minor actions like moving the eyes, or major activities like walking, become spasmodic as the muscles involved contract too much or too little and operate out of sequence. However, because the cerebellum is supplied by three major arteries on each side (see Chapter 7), there are many potential stroke syndromes for the medical assessment to consider. As I have said already, despite what I would call the gross symptoms that I displayed (vomiting and speech problems) during the first 24 hours, it was for a concern in connection with the medical assessment of my eyes that the doctors arranged the CT scan. I was lucky, because as obvious as my other symptoms were, they could have applied to any number of conditions that might have resulted in me being discharged from hospital without the scan and treatment. In a study entitled 'Can cerebellar infarctions be overlooked?' (Taycan *et al.* 2002, p.51), the researchers wrote: '...early diagnosis and treatment usually may save life and prevent catastrophic complications.'

Gill explained to us that, simply speaking, the clot had stopped the blood supply to some of the cells in this area of my brain, which then died. This was as opposed to a bleed in the brain itself, which would have been categorised as a *haemorrhagic stroke*. The physiology of these different causes of stroke is discussed in Chapter 6 'What Is a Stroke?'.

I was incredibly lucky, as a clot in this area of the brain can cause *hydrocephalus*, which can be very dangerous. It is not too uncommon for cerebellar stroke victims to spend time on a life support machine. In fact, a clot in the cerebellum is one of the few circumstances where an operation may be required to remove the clot, or even part of the cerebellum.

Haemorrhagic stroke occurs when a blood vessel in the brain bursts, spilling blood into the spaces surrounding the brain cells, or when a cerebral aneurysm ruptures. It is also called an intracranial haemorrhage.

Hydrocephalus is a condition in which cerebrospinal fluid accumulates in the skull and puts pressure on the brain tissue. Hydrocephalus is sometimes inaccurately referred to as 'water on the brain'. (See also Glossary.)

Gill told us that most of the tests I had undergone, and was still to undergo, were to try to establish where the clot had come from, and why it had formed. The good news was that lumbar puncture would not now be necessary as the reasons for my collapse were clear, even if the primary cause was not. She told us that since the results of the CT scan had been known I had been given a high daily dose of aspirin to disperse the clot and so prevent further damage. We were told that due to the medication the clot had probably already been dispersed during the previous days and it was likely that I was free from any immediate risk. She continued, saying that I would be advised to take aspirin for the rest of my life. I was aware of the internal bleeding associated with aspirin takers but immediately calculated that, for me, it was worth the risk. This potential stomach irritation must really be taken seriously and I discuss this in more detail in Chapter 10 'A Toolkit for Recovery and Prevention'.

Stroke and aspirin

Aspirin was the first drug to be produced in a laboratory and is now one of the most widely available and inexpensive of all drugs. The mechanism by which aspirin works in the treatment of heart attack and stroke is not completely understood. However, it is an antiplatelet drug that helps reduce platelet clumping, which can cause blockage in blood vessels.

The UK Stroke Association says that aspirin helps reduce the risk of a further stroke by as much as one third and may also help to prevent a heart attack. More than 20 million Americans reportedly use aspirin each day to prevent blood clots and reduce the risk of heart attack and stroke.

Aspirin like any medication has potential side-effects, including internal bleeding, stomach ulcers and even hearing loss or tinnitus, a ringing in the ears. To combat any side-effects aspirin should be taken with food.

Gill did not dwell on my inability to speak during the stroke. However, she explained that in my case it was due to a condition called *dysarthria*, which is common to those who have a stroke in the cerebellum. Dysarthria is very different from the other speech and language conditions associated with strokes, which include *dysphasia* and *dyspraxia of speech*. Eventually she presented me with more leaflets about strokes and left me with the appointment times when the physiotherapist and occupational therapist would be calling to see me. It is certainly not uncommon for several therapists to work with a stroke survivor. Research at the Mayo Clinic Stroke Centre (Wiebers 2001) reports that 50 per cent of individuals who survive an ischaemic stroke benefit from physical therapy, 40 per cent benefit from occupational therapy, and 15 per cent from speech therapy.

After visiting time was over I felt very much alone, possibly for the first time in my life. I decided to try to use that feeling to my advantage and just

Dysarthria is the inability to articulate clearly due to facial paralysis, which can produce weaknesses in co-ordination of the muscles of the face, tongue and throat. It can result from a stroke occurring in any one of several parts of the brain.

Dysphasia is a difficulty with understanding language generally.

Dyspraxia of speech is the partial loss of the ability to consistently pronounce words in individuals with normal muscle tone and co-ordination of the speech muscles.

let my unconscious mind lead my thoughts and moods. This is something I continued to let happen in the weeks and months that followed.

It was actually the term 'stroke', rather than the physiology of what had happened, that I had a problem accepting. I still had strong feelings of prejudice about 'who' a stroke victim was and as a consequence felt very far removed from the type of person who would have a stroke. Having spoken to Gill, and to some extent accepting that I had suffered a stroke, I then had a difficult few days coping emotionally when I was faced with seeing another patient who had also been admitted following a stroke. He was in a bed right opposite mine. He was a strong, athletic looking man in his fifties. My introduction to our new companion had been a few days earlier, watching him lying up in bed urinating over himself, grinning madly. He was unable to talk coherently at all at this stage, and this was the most recent of a series of strokes he had suffered in a very short space of time. The only word he said with any clarity was 'homosexuals', which he kept repeating frequently. It seemed to be the only word that he was able to use to communicate. In addition, he was constantly trying to get out of bed and began ripping the intravenous drip out of his arm, which resulted in a lot of blood on his bedding. This was disturbing for all of us and, again, did not help me to associate myself with the condition of stroke.

Frank, in the next bed to him, found the nights extremely distressing, and Ken, who was supposed to be resting, was getting in and out of bed to stop the new patient from falling out of bed. Eventually, the other stroke survivor in the ward had to be secured to the bed for his own safety. I spoke to the staff on Frank's behalf, who then allowed him to sleep with his curtain closed and also checked on us all more frequently.

This period was one of the most difficult times for me. Ken, Frank and most of the others were in the ward with heart problems. For the most part, they all looked reasonably well and were mentally coherent. Now I was faced, literally, with someone else who had had a stroke. I was still unable to look in a mirror, and yet opposite me was an image of just how close I had been to suffering more damage or, worse, an image of what the future might hold. I stared across the ward at him, still thinking that stroke as an affliction was remote from me. How was it possible that it had happened to me? In truth, this experience and the associated insight as to what the future might have in store for me is something I still can't quite come to terms with, and something I find very upsetting. I do not apply these worries just to me. It has got to the stage that every time I see someone smoking, a very public and well-known health risk in terms of strokes, I think to myself – if only you knew! Why are you doing that to yourself? Don't contribute to giving yourself a stroke! It could happen! I was doing very little wrong, and it happened to me!

It was during one hospital visiting session that I felt overwhelmed by everything for the first time. My mother and Anne were with me as usual. Mark had called up to the ward to give his grandfather a rest. Paul had arrived to check up on my progress, and so too did one of my close friends who had heard that I was unwell from a third party. The new visitor, Martyn, was the former PE teacher of the male nurse. Martyn and I had become friends after encouraging some fierce competitiveness and rivalry between our school teams. Slightly older than me, Martyn was one of the most gifted sportsmen I had ever seen. We went to fitness classes together, played golf and skied together regularly and even learnt to scuba dive together.

Remembering the good memories, all involving physical activity, proved to be very unsettling and I started to feel quite daunted by the future.

Chapter 4

Taking Control

Returning home

Many stroke survivors are hospitalised for months, and individual circumstances will dictate when they can return home. Other stroke survivors are not admitted to hospital at all. Every hospital has its own procedures, which will have been agreed by a number of agencies, for the discharge of patients. However, the priority will always be for a patient to leave when it is safe, and he or she is fit, to do so.

I was discharged only after I was able to walk short distances unaided (the physiotherapist had worked with me on the ward and the stairs) and when Karen, the occupational therapist, had assessed me in the Occupational Therapy Unit (OTU). As my circumstances meant that I would be able to be supervised at home, I was declared to be safe from risk of an accident in the house. This was despite some slowness, confusion and clumsiness exhibited during the assessment. In the OTU, while trying to co-ordinate my hands to plug in the kettle (one of the more straightforward tests!), the lead got tangled with the telephone, which I managed to rip completely off the wall. Nevertheless, I was ready to go home.

On reflection, I don't feel that I established a bond with anyone at the hospital apart from Ken. As we lay on our beds, all social and age barriers had been broken down by the very fact that we shared the same emotions. We were both ill, we were both apprehensive as to the future and we both needed someone to share our anxiety with.

My home environment and my level of mobility was such that I did not require any modified equipment. However, I am sure that I would have been given a great deal of advice and support should this have been necessary. Contact details for the Disabled Living Centres Council and other organisations who can offer advice on such things is available in Appendix II.

By the time I returned home, I was taking two tablets daily in addition to the aspirin and *simvastatin*. Although acetaminophen, ibuprofen, naproxyn sodium and ketoprofen are good drugs for pain and fever, as is aspirin, only aspirin has demonstrated a beneficial effect for heart attack and stroke. Simvastatin, on the other hand, is used to reduce the amount of *cholesterol* and certain fatty substances in the blood. I was prescribed this because one of the blood tests had shown that my cholesterol was slightly higher than the optimum level suggested by experts.

Simvastatin can lower cholesterol by up to 20 per cent and inhibits the production of cholesterol by the liver. It lowers overall blood cholesterol as well as low-density lipoprotein cholesterol levels. The lowering of the level of cholesterol and fats in the blood may help to prevent a further stroke, heart disease, angina and heart attacks. Side-effects from simvastatin are not common, but include stomach pain or cramps, liver irritation, wind, diarrhoea, constipation, heartburn, headache, blurred vision, dizziness, rash or itching, muscle pain, muscle tenderness, or weakness with or without a fever.

Cholesterol is a soft, waxy substance found among the lipids (fats) in the bloodstream and in all the body's cells. Cholesterol is an important part of a healthy body as it is used to form cell membrane, various hormones, bile salts and vitamin D. People get cholesterol in their blood in two ways. It is produced naturally in the liver, and it is ingested through food. Foods from animals (especially egg yolks, meat, poultry, fish, seafood and whole-milk dairy products) contain it, but foods from plants (fruits, vegetables, grains, nuts and seeds) do not. The body (typically) makes all the cholesterol it needs, and so it does not need to be consumed. Nevertheless, we do consume it, and saturated fatty acids are the main contributory factor in raising blood cholesterol. While some of this excess dietary cholesterol is removed from the body through the liver, by keeping the dietary intake of saturated fats low, individuals could significantly lower their dietary cholesterol intake.

Cholesterol and other fats can't dissolve in the blood. They have to be transported to and from the cells by special carriers called lipoproteins. There are several kinds, but the ones relevant in this context are low-density lipoprotein (LDL) and high-density lipoprotein (HDL).

LDL is the major cholesterol carrier in the blood. If too much LDL cholesterol circulates in the blood, it can slowly build up in the walls of the arteries feeding the heart and brain. Together with other substances LDL can cause atherosclerosis. A clot that forms near this plaque can block the blood flow to part of the heart muscle and cause a heart attack, or to the blood flow to part of the brain, resulting in a stroke. A high level of LDL cholesterol reflects an increased risk of heart disease and is sometimes called 'bad' cholesterol. Simply speaking, lower levels of LDL cholesterol reflect a lower risk of heart disease and strokes.

HDL carries one third to one fourth of blood cholesterol. HDL carries cholesterol away from the arteries back to the liver, where it is passed from the body. Some experts believe HDL removes excess cholesterol from plaque and actually slows down plaque growth. HDL cholesterol is known as 'good' cholesterol because a high HDL level seems to protect against heart attack.

'Your cholesterol is not classed as high,' Dr Evans had explained. 'It is just that in the context of you having had a stroke we will take action to control and lower it. This should be supplemented by a dietary review. To be honest, if you had had your cholesterol checked last week, before having the stroke, you would not have been prescribed anything.'

Nevertheless, at home, I decided it was time to pay more attention to what I was putting into my body at meal times and, more importantly, between meals through snacking. I did not eat a truly bad diet before the stroke, but it was time to improve. I had been eating school dinners every day at work and Anne and I ate microwave meals too regularly – as we were often too tired to cook and prepare fresh food. I illustrate how my diet has changed in Chapter 10 'A Toolkit for Recovery and Prevention' and provide useful guidelines for anyone wishing to plan a healthy diet. Dietary advice can be very confusing, especially as some diets are related more to weight loss than health. On the other hand, there is still much to discover and the effect of diet is a complex issue. With regard to cholesterol, which I also discuss in Chapter 10 in terms of diet, unlike many other possible contributory factors of stroke it has the advantage that it is measurable and treatable. With this in mind, I gladly accepted that I would be taking a second tablet for the rest of my life, which would supplement my diet. Whatever the cause of my stroke would prove to be, I was determined that all preventive measures were worth taking. As I frequently said to the students on the sports injuries course I taught, 'Prevention is far better than cure!'

As I planned what I was putting into my body with more detail than I had done for some years, I wondered if most people were prepared to spend as much on making the inside healthy and last a long time as they were spending on making the outside look good. Did the spending on good, fresh, healthy food and supplements match the spending on tanning, or on toiletries such as creams, lotions, shampoo, conditioner, gel and perfume or aftershave? Sadly, I am confident that the money spent on plastic surgery (I refer to procedures such as botox and implants to lips undertaken for vanity, and not those procedures undertaken for medical reasons such as reconstructive surgery) by many people far outweighs that which they spend on eating healthily.

The first few days at home involved turning the phone off and sitting. I was too tired to talk and not strong enough to move much. Still, word of an illness or event like stroke spreads quickly and I reluctantly had to speak to some people on the phone. I soon became used to one of the most unhelpful comments of all: 'You are the last person I would ever have expected to suffer a stroke.' I still haven't thought of an appropriate response to this statement. As conversations went on I was invariably asked, 'Why did it happen?' While this is asked after a serious injury, Anne pointed out that this is an unusual question in terms of serious illness. You don't ask someone with kidney failure 'Why has that happened then?' or with breast cancer 'Do they know why you have that?' So, when asked this question I just repeated what the stroke nurse told me. I did not know why it had happened and, in fact, it is not unusual for the cause of stroke never to be known in younger individuals.

In between visits and phone calls Anne had to go to work, which was hard for her. When you have a class of 30 pupils in front of you there is nowhere to hide. You have to give it your all. Teachers who do not give a lesson their full attention are found out. There are no moments when you can afford to indulge in private thoughts or have a lapse in concentration. Any moments of weakness will be spotted and capitalised on by certain individuals in the group. Furthermore, as we worked in the same school, Anne was constantly reminded of me, and our situation, from the moment she began the day by having to travel in with someone else, through to enquiries from individual colleagues, pupils and parents. I dreaded colleagues from school wanting to visit, as I had no interest in how the school was surviving without me. I expect my colleagues would have inevitably paid lip service to how I was being missed, but I knew that the truth was if I was never to go back it would not matter. Someone else would simply fill my shoes. While I was not concerned with work in terms of the institution, for the first few months I was unable to forget about work and felt that I had to make an immediate decision about whether I was going to return. This was contrary to the messages coming from my head teacher and governors who could not have been more supportive or sympathetic. However, this issue of work became a major problem and cause of anxiety as the months progressed, as I will explain later.

During my stay in hospital, I had arranged with the occupational therapist that someone would be with me at home for the first few weeks. My mother duly came around every day. She presented me with lunch and continued her interest in my 'bowel movement' until the lactulose eventually worked. I was relieved that no 'straining' was necessary and wasted no time in presenting her with an update!

I was just about able to manage the stairs, although coming down was far harder than going up, and I limited their use to twice a day. I went down them in the morning and up them at night. In between, I really just sat. The feeling of dizziness was still with me every day, and I was unsteady and unsafe on my feet. In addition, I was still taking regular painkillers for the headache.

After a few weeks, I was able to read for short periods of time. I tentatively reached for the stroke information left by the doctor the morning I was told that I had had a stroke. The literature included *Stroke in Younger Adults*, *Driving After a Stroke*, *Aspirin and Stroke*, *How to Reduce Your Risk of a Stroke*, *Stroke: Questions and Answers*, *Diet and Stroke*, *Depression after Stroke* and the intriguingly titled *Sex after Stroke*. I read some of the literature and actually felt sick with worry. I must be honest, while the care in hospital was good, I felt very much left alone when discharged from hospital and this added to feelings of insecurity. I am not alone in feeling like this, as many stroke survivors I have spoken to while writing this book volunteered that they felt the same. Nevertheless, very gradually I stuck with it and eventually learned more about strokes. Initially, I was able to read these booklets for just a few minutes without dizziness, losing concentration, or just plain fear. However, as the days went by I controlled my fear, and my concentration and ability to read increased.

During this time, I ended up back at my doctor's as an emergency on one occasion. Anne made me go because throughout the day, but on a very much milder level, I felt some of the symptoms I had felt during the stroke. Fortunately, everything seemed to be in order and I started to feel better during the night.

Making progress

'What we need to do is practise taking time out to be human beings rather than human doings.'

Cary Cooper, Professor of Psychology and Health, Lancaster University

Feeling safe at home, I quickly became an avid watcher of daytime TV. I became enthralled by stories of love triangles, threesomes, adultery, insecurity, drugs, alcohol, family break-ups and lie detector tests. Generally, I found that visitors intruded on my state of fatigue and confusion, and I actively continued to deter them from visiting. Anne supported me with this, but this was something I think my mother had difficulty in accepting, as she had to explain to various family members and friends that I did not want to see anyone. Nevertheless, I think that this time was vitally important for me. Initially, I needed time to be alone and to try to work through the process of denial and acceptance before I could identify a strategy for improvement. However, some people took it upon themselves just to turn up – including people I hadn't seen for years. I said all the right things, including what they wanted to hear, and they left happy enough. My mother couldn't win, as later, when the initial months had passed, I did not want visitors to make a special trip to see me because the inevitable focus would have been on my stroke whereas I then wanted to focus on continuing to improve and preparing for the future. I suppose, at times like this, following a major life event, we should all remember that behaviour is not a definition of who the person is. Rather, behaviour is the result of an internal interpretation and response to a variety of stimuli – some of which will be experiences.

The components that make up a normal daily routine were tiring, and at times I failed to motivate myself to complete them. I did not want to go through the routine of showering every day. I didn't want to answer the door. I didn't want to have to initiate any conversation with anyone. I did not even want to make conversation with my parents during their visits. I generally looked the same as before, apart from the fact that I refused to have a haircut. This was strange as my curly hair grows out not down, and my usual routine was to cut it every three weeks. It was three months before I actually made it to a barber's chair to have it cut. Perhaps significantly, I went to a new barber where I was anonymous and did not have to explain why my routine had been broken. I simply could not face the endless questions I associated with a trip to have a haircut: 'I haven't seen you for a while, have I?', 'Oh, your hair has grown, have you been on holiday?' or 'Are you going out tonight?' Anne's favourite question is always 'How's your hair been?'

For a time I was concerned about my eyesight and the health of my eyes. I had changed optician's only months before the stroke and, unlike the barber or dentist, I did not have an established relationship with him. Significantly, I had an appointment within two weeks of being at home and was able to attend.

'If you hadn't told me about the stroke I wouldn't have known from your eyes,' he stated, very reassuringly.

Similarly, I was due for an appointment at the dentist as I had cracked a tooth in hospital. I had never been concerned with trips to the dentist and over a 20 year period had established a friendly relationship with mine. My dentist, also a keen skier, and I would always update each other about any new resorts we had visited, or that we could recommend. Suddenly, I did not want to go to see him. I did not want to answer the question 'How have you been since you were in last?' I did not want to recount what had happened. I did not want sympathy and I certainly did not want to see another shocked expression on anyone's face. However, I could not simply change dentists like barbers. I was unable to be anonymous when in the dentist's chair and it was over five months before I was ready to face him. It wasn't too bad after all, and he advised me to start using an electric toothbrush, which did make cleaning my teeth very much easier.

I had been home from hospital a week when I had a visit from Anne's brother, a senior nurse who has worked extensively with plastic surgery and burns victims. He and I have always got on well. He is a keen sportsman, and he once accompanied me on a school ski trip. On this occasion he made me laugh with a story about an inebriated man who required surgery after getting his penis stuck in a letter box – the events that led up to him deciding to engage in such an activity probably contribute to an interesting story on their own. We went for a walk, and with his support I walked some yards to the end of the road despite some difficulties with visual perception, balance and a strange feeling in my left leg and foot. These feelings remained for some months, and compounded by difficulties with balance and an affected gait meant that uneven ground proved problematic for some time; and although I only fell on a few occasions, I was regularly twisting an ankle.

Fatigue proved to be a major problem and I was actually waking up as tired as when I had gone to bed. This caused Anne a lot of distress at the time. My breathing and twitching concerned her, and she often thought that I was having another stroke! In fact, for some time I was reliving the actual stroke in my dreams. The brain has an amazing way of both consciously and unconsciously recreating experiences resulting in a physiological response. For example, people who, like me, are not comfortable around snakes shiver just at the thought of them, and we all salivate at thought of our favourite food. However, on these nocturnal occasions I was reliving the stroke and the helplessness I had felt. So Anne developed a routine of gently rubbing my brow and whispering that I was all right until my breathing quietened down. Still, I woke up each morning feeling shattered.

Unfortunately, fatigue after a stroke does not go away after a good night's sleep. Unlike many of the other repercussions of stroke, it is one of the least known effects. It can be truly overwhelming, can interfere with some rehabilitation programmes and can actually be more of a hindrance to a stroke survivor leading a full life than some physical deficits. There are several theories about the onset of post-stroke fatigue, which include both the physical damage to the brain itself and the effect the trauma has on the chemicals that are released into the bloodstream. It may be that patients who suffer post-stroke fatigue the most are the older ones, who were in fact in poor health before the stroke. The feeling of fatigue I felt was not constant. It would appear and build up without warning, manifest itself with a physical and mental lack of energy and then pass after a few days. I have included some general tips which may help with this issue in the box 'Dealing with post-stroke fatigue', adapted from the Stroke Association's *Stroke News* (Lantin 2003).

Dealing with post-stroke fatigue

- Keep active in the day and develop a routine for preparing to sleep at night.
- Discuss with your doctor the option of a sleeping tablet.
- If necessary, rest for short periods in the day.
- Try the 'power nap' methods to daytime sleeping (see Chapter 10).
- Develop an exercise routine and consult with your physiotherapist to ensure that fatigue-fighting exercises are included.
- Perhaps join a t'ai chi or chikung class (see Chapter 10).
- Set realistic goals for each day.
- Celebrate all achievement.
- Incorporate positive language into your thoughts, goal setting and celebration of achievement.
- Ask healthcare professionals for help.

One evening, one of my closest friends, also called Andy, telephoned. We have always kept in touch by phone on a monthly basis. I had specifically told Anne not to phone him or he would have dropped everything to travel to see me. He had married Lisa, an American girl, several years earlier, and after conscientiously performing my duties as best man at the wedding, Anne and I are now godparents to their children.

'I've got some news, I'm off into hospital tomorrow,' he began in his usual, jovial way.

'What's up?' I asked, and was momentarily worried about someone else.

'I'm having a vasectomy,' he said.

I was relieved that it was nothing serious.

'I can beat that,' I said. 'I've not long come out of hospital.'

'Why?'

'I've had a stroke,' I replied. The phrase was starting to become easier to say.

There was silence on the phone.

'Andy? You all right?' I asked.

Within a week, and post vasectomy, he was with me, and it was really good to see him. Getting directly to the point, he said, 'Right, you had better consider how you were pre-stroke is probably no longer the norm for you. Enjoy the memories and make the most of what the new norm might be. In time they may overlap more than you think they could right now. Just get on with life.'

There it was, as simple as that.

With the serious chat over we decided to go for a short walk. We really must have looked very funny to other pedestrians. I shuffled, unsteady as usual, while he, suffering some discomfort after his surgery, walked like he was a cowboy wearing a nappy. As we walked, he told me of his operation – in great detail!

Not everyone seemed to understand how I was feeling like Andy did. I heard expressions of sympathy, words of encouragement and genuine enquiries after my health, but people were unable truly to understand the colossal consequences and turmoil a stroke victim must face. I realised that people generally accepted that a brain injury could change thoughts and memories, but I thought that most would have difficulty understanding that it also changes emotions. However, I was starting to develop an acceptance, albeit an uneasy one, of what had happened to me. As the teacher, and world famous sports broadcaster, Bill McLaren wrote in his autobiography, 'All manner of things are thrown at us in this world, and we have to accept that our lives will be a pot-pourri of good times and bad' (2004, p.288).

My first visit to the newsagents on my own, a few weeks later, felt like quite an adventure. For the most part, I was on edge that the unexpected approach of someone may cause me to startle and fall over. It was also strange to think that other people were going about their daily business, completely unaware of the sheer nervous excitement I felt at going to the shop. However, the trip was a success and gradually I grew in confidence. At home, I was still walking into doorframes and unable to put pants on while standing up without losing my balance, which Anne found very funny. She repeatedly referred to me as 'Norman', after the British comedy actor Norman Wisdom, whose trademark was his ability to 'fall'. I did not take offence.

However, balance problems can be a serious issue for stroke survivors. In addition to the feelings of nausea and dizziness, falls and fall-related injuries are among the most common complications after a stroke, leading to a real lack of confidence. Balance is controlled by a number of different systems in the body, and a stroke can injure one of these systems, injure the nerves that send messages to the balance centres in the brain, injure one of the balance centres in the brain itself (as in my case), or affect balance by paralysing one side of the body, which in turn leads to balance problems. I have included some general tips which may help with this issue in the box 'Dealing with balance problems', adapted from the Stroke Association's *Stroke News* (Stroke Association 2004).

I began walking to the newsagents on a daily basis. I considered it important to give the activity a purpose. I set about collecting tokens from our daily newspaper. Anne was not as impressed as I expected her to be when after collecting 18 different tokens and sending a small cheque, a 'Cottage Garden Set Flower Bulbs' arrived in the post. Unfortunately, the big prizes, the £100,000, the holiday villas and the cars, all went elsewhere.

As the weeks went by, I concentrated exclusively on getting better. With my father's daily help I was walking non-stop for 40 minutes a day. My balance was not what it had been before the stroke, and I was unhappy with the way my left leg and foot felt. Most people did not notice, but some friends enquired whether I was 'dragging' my left leg. My foot felt like it was not making contact with the ground and I was walking on air. In retrospect, I feel sorry for what my father went through at this time. I can be fairly quiet at the best of times, but now the fact that I had had a stroke was sinking in I was more quiet than usual. I wanted to walk but did not want to talk.

Dealing with balance problems

Avoiding a fall

- Flooring: be aware of rugs, carpets and uneven floors.
- Footwear: wear comfortable, supporting shoes and slippers.
- Reaching high: be aware of high shelves and cupboards which could result in overbalancing.
- Reaching low: be aware of low shelves and cupboards which could result in overbalancing.
- Lighting: dim lighting increases the risk of falling.
- Night-time bathroom visits: leave a light on in readiness.
- Hearing aid: wear one if necessary.
- Grab rails: talk to the occupational therapist about any house adaptations.

Physiotherapy

- Exercises: your physiotherapist will advise the most suitable exercises which will address the individual problems with the balance systems.
- Safety: exercises sould be practised in a safe environment.
- Stationary balance: issues relating to sitting balance should be addressed early (this may extend to dressing and reaching).
- Transferring: the issue of moving from a chair (to a bed or toilet) should be addressed.
- Dynamic: issues relating to whole-body movement (walking) could be included.

I became reasonably pleased with my physical progress, and despite overwhelming feelings of fatigue I realised that I would only continue to progress if I did more. I decided to examine and apply the 'principles of training' that I had taught to my PE classes, which are explained in Chapter 10 'A Toolkit for Recovery and Prevention'.

As we walked around Cardiff's Roath Park, just down the road from where I live, we would regularly see people walking their dogs. I soon remembered a scheme that Anne and I had wanted to get involved in for some time, but due to the demands of work had never made definite enquiries about. Several months earlier, on a rare trip to the supermarket without me, Anne had met a lady with a Labrador dog and got into conversation. Anne learnt that although the lady was not blind herself, the dog was in fact a guide dog. She simply provided a boarding service for guide dogs. Now the time seemed right, and eventually I decided to go online to make enquiries about the scheme. I had avoided the computer in the weeks since returning from hospital as I could not face the emails, many from friends around the world, which would have been sent before I had had the stroke; or worse, subsequent enquiries as to why I had not sent a message back. Initially, I avoided my 'Inbox' and used the internet to contact the Guide Dogs for the Blind Association (UK). Soon, an application form arrived and the process began. Within a week our references had been taken up, something friends seemed to find hilarious, and I prepared for the 'home visit'. A Guide Dogs for the Blind dog trainer arrived. She checked the suitability of the house, our garden and our motives for signing up. We were soon listed to provide board for working dogs whose owners were going on holiday or into hospital, or to provide a home for dogs in training.

Lessons in psychology

I soon came to realise that, psychologically, the stroke had really changed me. Since the stroke, I had given virtually no thought to my job, to the people I worked with and children I taught. The significance of this is hard to explain. I did not work with materialistic commodities. I did not meet endless sales targets. I interacted, on one level or other, with over 750 individuals every day. To push them to the back of my mind so quickly and withdraw into my simplified life to the extent that I did was a new feeling for me. However, I was soon faced with a minor confrontation when I found myself in a situation with my bank. I had cause to complain but was scared to pick up the telephone to do it. As I stared at the phone, dwelling on the situation, I thought back to just a couple of years earlier when, on a trip to New York, I thought nothing of going on my own to a world famous jujutsu gym that trained professional full-contact fighters and putting my body and pride on the line by training with them. Now, I was unable to pick up the phone to make a simple complaint. When Anne arrived home from work she found me on edge, pacing about. I confessed to her that I was scared at the thought of talking to the bank and was almost at the point of tears when I had tried to do it. This was a very odd feeling. Previously I had always rather enjoyed a good opportunity to complain to someone! With tips from my father I had successfully taken on the council and various national companies. I felt scared and vulnerable at the thought of any confrontation. Given my previous level of confidence, my previous experience and my profession, this was a source of concern to me.

The word 'confidence' is actually derived from two Latin words – *cum* (with) and *fides* (faith). It is probable that confidence grows from the assurance of previous positive experience. Despite the abundance of positive experiences I had had in my life, most had become consumed, at least for several months, by the experience of stroke. I then became anxious about the fact that I was anxious, and, for the first time, realised why the request to 'protect us from all anxiety' found its way into the Catholic mass, after the Lord's Prayer. I had come to the point where I was almost being controlled by my anxiety.

The characteristics of anxiety are that it is distressing and its sources are indefinite. It is common after a sudden event like a stroke because it's an event that is not planned for, and in some circumstances not even expected. I found it a strange emotion, and I generally felt a nervousness and vulnerability about something that I could not really identify. It was just a feeling that something was imminent. In my case, the anxiety was directed at the future as I tried to predict things that might happen. Clinical psychologists often believe that anxiety is one of the most distressing emotions that people feel, and problems such as phobias, panic attacks, post-traumatic stress disorder and obsessive compulsive disorder, as well as generalised anxiety disorder, are each associated with it. Most people who are anxious are aware of the physical symptoms (tension, sweating, increased heart rate, headaches and even breathing difficulties) but perhaps are not so aware of how the physical, behavioural and thinking aspects of life are so closely related. Anxiety is actually a natural response to help cope with a given situation. However, too much anxiety interferes with good coping, and for a time the feelings perhaps influenced how I coped.

Even with stroke survivors with a significant degree of physical recovery, studies have shown that a degree of social isolation is still evident (Gordon *et al.* 2004). After my experience, I can fully appreciate why this is so.

As I was fighting off daily feelings of anxiety, which at times became feelings of self-pity, I heard about the book *My Year Off: Rediscovering Life after a Stroke*, written by journalist and stroke survivor Robert McCrum. I was able to read reasonably well by this time and so got hold of a copy from the library, which was within my walking range. Unfortunately, I wasn't emotionally ready to read it when I did. The book sparked off different emotions. I felt guilty that his stroke left him with greater physical difficulties than I had. I felt envious that he was able to see some of the country's top medical specialists, having private seminars and meetings, while I waited three months for my first appointment with a consultant after being discharged from hospital. I was unhappy that he spoke of his private room in hospital when I had to deal with some patients dying around me, and lying directly opposite someone who may have been showing me what lay in store for me. I got angry with him for seemingly 'walking into' a new job, and even scoffed at the fact that despite all this he still contemplated suicide.

Instead of stopping with McCrum's book, I then read *My Stroke of Luck*, written by Kirk Douglas after his stroke. I remembered how I thought of Kirk during the first hours in hospital. However, this book, too, also made me angry. Kirk obviously did not have to worry about his finances like I did. He spoke of his housekeeper and largely idyllic life with his dogs. He wrote of travelling in private planes, and of his wonderful family, and yet he too had contemplated suicide. He said that he searched his mind for nice memories that he could enjoy and focus on before going to sleep. I found myself thinking, 'How would you have liked it if your stroke had happened when you were 37 years old? About the time you filmed *The Juggler*. A whole 15 years before you made *Gunfight at the OK Corral* or *The Vikings*! How depressed would you have felt then?' I even spent the time looking up his filmography to see what he was doing when he was my age, so I could complain even more to myself. I realised that I was becoming bitter. It was the first time in my life I had ever felt emotions like it.

Nevertheless, I tried Kirk's tips for going to sleep, as this was also hard for me, with the nights being the worst part of the daily cycle. In hospital, I had been so mentally and physically drained by everything that I slept reasonably well. I had managed to block out the groans from the other patients — some of whom unfortunately died from their afflictions. Now, in the comfort of my own bed, I kept reliving the time of the stroke and I remembered the fear I had then that I might have remained in that physical state for the rest of my life. I often wondered what was worse. Being completely disabled by a stroke, or trying to care for a loved one who had. I went to sleep most nights wondering if another stroke would strike during the night. When I would wake up, the anxiety started immediately as I felt the need to check that I had full use of each limb and my facial muscles before I tried to get out of bed.

Unfortunately it was at this time I came across a newspaper headline, which stated that strokes double the risk of *Alzheimer's disease*. This was a difficult thought to deal with. I already held the belief (this was just a gut feeling and nothing that I had ever researched) that teachers were more susceptible to Alzheimer's disease than other people. I had witnessed first-hand the rapid deterioration of a friend and colleague to the illness within months of finishing teaching early in order to enjoy his retirement. I can honestly say that due to the illness, he did not enjoy any quality retirement time before his death. As I read more, things went from bad to worse and I became more insecure, eventually 'discovering' *vascular dementia*. In the case of vascular dementia, the main means of prevention are thought to be the same as for stroke disease, namely the control of high blood pressure, together with aspirin tablets. I felt a moment's relief that I was already contributing to the prevention of this with my little aspirin tablet.

Alzheimer's disease is a degenerative disease of the brain (dementia) from which there is no recovery. Very much like stroke, each case has unique circumstances. Slowly the disease attacks nerve cells in all parts of the cortex of the brain, as well as some surrounding structures, thereby impairing a person's abilities to govern emotions, recognise errors and patterns, co-ordinate movement, and remember. Eventually, an afflicted person loses all memory and mental functioning. Unless effective methods for prevention and treatment are developed, experts believe that Alzheimer's will reach epidemic proportions by the middle of this century. The risk of developing dementia increases with age – the percentage of people in the population with dementia doubles every five years over the age of 65. Dementia is the fourth most common cause of death after heart disease, cancer and stroke.

Vascular dementia is a group of disorders in which brain cells are damaged by abnormal blood circulation to the brain. It may take the form of multiple 'mini-strokes', leading to a step-by-step deterioration. Or in other cases the small blood vessels become narrowed, leading to a progressive loss of blood supply.

The next thing I discovered was that recurrent strokes are frequent. Approximately 25 per cent of people who recover from a first stroke will have another stroke within five years. The risk of a recurrent stroke is actually greatest right after a stroke, with the risk decreasing with time. About 3 per cent of stroke patients will have another stroke within 30 days of their first stroke and one third of recurrent strokes take place within two years of the first stroke. The recurrent stroke is a major contributor to stroke disability and death, with the risk of severe disability or death from stroke increasing with each stroke recurrence.

So for a while I waited for the second stroke, which took my mind off the long-term worry of Alzheimer's disease and dementia. I think that I harboured some fears that perhaps I hadn't been told the truth about the stroke and that next time it would be worse. The unpredictability of what I interpreted my situation to be was, at this time, exhausting. Furthermore, the fear of a second, and worse, stroke was very potent.

As I continued to find out more about strokes, I came across the startling statistic that approximately 50 per cent of all stroke victims experience clinical depression, which made me feel even worse! Depression is quite common following a brain injury. In some cases it is caused by physical damage to the brain, while in other cases it is an emotional reaction to injury and disability. It is estimated that half of those who survive a stroke will experience depression at some stage in the first few years. Depression does not recognise age or gender. It can develop immediately after a stroke, or some months later, and can vary from being relatively mild to very severe. Apparently, those who suffer depression as a result of their stroke do not appear to recover as well as those who are unaffected by it. It can last for just a few months, or for years. One stroke survivor and sufferer of depression himself wrote 'depression, although frightening, is never permanent' (Hinds 2000). However, it has been reported that depression itself may increase the risk of stroke (Jonas and Mussolino 2000).

I decided to try to keep some structure to my day and apply strategies to combat this. These strategies are expanded on in Chapter 10 'A Toolkit for Recovery and Prevention'.

While I was worrying about depression, I also found time to worry that I was going to bleed heavily if I cut myself. I had always regarded myself as a good 'clotter', and I became queasy thinking of the effect that my daily dose of aspirin was going to have. I knew that I was being irrational, but Anne still had to buy me a spray for cuts that 'seals the wound' in order to keep me quiet.

During the first months at home I still suffered from fairly disabling dizzy spells. For the most part, such feelings of vertigo were consistent with the damage to my cerebellum. On the rare occasion, it may have been due to fluctuations in my blood pressure as I conducted my investigative crusade into the world of medicine. More than one visitor a day left me feeling exhausted. Some, I learned later, told Anne that I was looking far from my usual robust self. Meanwhile, Anne was phoning home every day and would worry if I failed to answer.

I did, however, manage a trip to the cinema with Paul and Mark, as we are all movie fans. I suppose there are no surprises that we saw films rife with action and martial arts – namely, *The Last Samurai*, starring Tom Cruise, and Quentin Tarantino's *Kill Bill 2*, with Uma Thurman. I also had a couple of walks with Bill, a cousin's husband who was very kind and visited on my terms, when it was convenient to me, and not just because he was passing and felt that it was his duty to call in. Andy and some of my other close friends reappeared and insisted I leave the house to watch the international rugby matches held at Cardiff. Nevertheless, 2004 was the first year for almost 20 years when I had not made it to all the Wales home international games in Cardiff.

On such trips, I occasionally met people I knew who were ignorant of the fact that I had had a stroke. In response to their enquiries about why I was not in work, or when they gave the general greeting 'How are you?', I found myself failing to tell them that I had had a stroke. Rather mysteriously, I just said my health had been poor and I did not know when I would be returning to work. In fact, though I met my next-door neighbour twice during this time, I didn't tell him that I had had a stroke. Then one night, out of the blue, he knocked at our door, so I invited him in.

'I'm sorry to disturb you both,' he said, and referring to his wife, 'but we are really worried about you. We want you to know we are just next door if ever you need us. I've called in for our benefit really, can I ask you what's wrong?'

'I have had a stroke,' I said. 'I did mean to say, but I didn't want to alarm you.'

'I wasn't sure what it was. I saw that your face was drooping a bit and I thought you might have had a breakdown. My brother actually had a stroke. He's older than you and made a good recovery.'

We talked for a while, and on his way out he said something, which I found strangely reassuring and Anne found hilarious: 'I'm relieved,' he said. 'At least it's nothing serious!'

I do not think that I was in denial of the stroke, but it was a major life event such that was not in my nature to share with other people.

Rehabilitation for a stroke victim is generally designed to help the individual cope with the permanent effects of the stroke that are the result of the brain damage. It is usually co-ordinated between healthcare professionals after any spontaneous recovery has ceased. I decided that I was in a strong position to help myself and the methods I employed are developed in Chapter 10. I came to realise that thoughts and habits that limit your beliefs and actions can be as devastating in the way that positive and resourceful thoughts can be empowering.

As time went by and I started to become more positive, I thought back to Kirk Douglas. When he received his Academy Lifetime Achievement Award in person it was in front of an audience of two thousand and an estimated billion watching on TV. Eventually, I read his book a second time and better appreciated the insight with which it was written. One particular phrase that stayed with me was his belief that the world is filled with people who have suffered from one misfortune or another, and that the only thing that sets one apart from the rest is the desire and attempt to help others. While reading the book again, I spotted something that I had missed the first time as a result of my anger and bitterness. I was not the only one who could not look in the mirror. Kirk, too, could not face seeing himself for some time after his stroke (I quickly scanned through Robert McCrum's book, and again found that he was also unable to look in the mirror the week after his stroke).

Nevertheless, despite feeling a little more positive, I continued to waste a lot of nervous energy contemplating what the future would hold. I soon had an appointment with Dr Shetty, my new consultant at the Department of Integrated Medicine, University Hospital for Wales. Prior to this appointment I was unsure as to what I would be told. I was sure that I could not do my old job. I knew I wouldn't be able to teach physical education as I had done before. I didn't know whether I would be able to cope with the pressures of the other responsibilities I had before, or even those associated with simply teaching. I didn't know if I even wanted to go back to having the responsibilities of my old job. I was convinced that I should not ignore what had happened and simply go back to work as a matter of course. To me, even the word 'back' in this context implied that I would not be making the most of the opportunities having the stroke may have presented by allowing me to take stock, slow down and think. I just had to figure out what those opportunities were. The appointment went well, and Dr Shetty inspired me with confidence. He confirmed that my heart was strong and my arteries were clear. Some physical tests showed that my balance had improved, as had my co-ordination. Generally speaking, he encouraged me to keep up the light-to-moderate exercise, such as walking, that I had already started. However, he said that isometric exercises (i.e. where the muscle has been contracted, or is tense, but its length remains constant) should be avoided. Isometric exercise can rapidly raise blood pressure for the duration of the exercise, which is of course a risk factor for strokes. Unfortunately, lots of the physical training I enjoyed until this time had included isometric muscle work.

At the end of the consultation Dr Shetty told me that I was making progress and should not be concerned about having a second stroke as a result of the first one. While he stated that the cause of my stroke may well remain unknown, he was still prepared to conduct further tests to try to establish what actually caused it. In fact, in a subsequent appointment he stated that he believed my stroke was due to a tear and bleed (also known as shearing or dissection) in one of the vertebral arteries, known as vertebral arterial dissection (VAD), which is explained more fully in Chapter 8 'The Stroke: Signs, Symptoms and Causes'. Such a dissection can be the result of a traumatic movement or inflamed arteries, which are often grouped under the collective name of vasculitis. Vasculitis can be caused by a diverse range of contributory factors including syphilis, meningitis, rheumatoid arthritis, lupus and cocaine use. We discussed some of these issues (specifically, rheumatoid arthritis and lupus) and Dr Shetty stated there is often no apparent cause of the dissection in young adults. However, he remained interested in the fact that I had had a head and neck ache for some days before the stroke. Research has suggested that headache and neck pain are important warning symptoms of dissection, occurring in up to two thirds of patients hours, days and sometimes weeks before a stroke (Taycan *et al.* 2002). Apparently, in general terms, problems with the carotid arteries lead to a cerebral stroke, while problems with the vertebral arteries lead to a cerebellar stroke. Because VAD can be attributed to leaning back while getting your hair washed, it is also known as 'beauty parlour syndrome', which is ironic given my lack of any daily beauty regime. In my case, none of these were obvious causes – perhaps it just happened.

Following these consultations, it was hard to come to terms with what had been said. It was hard to be emotionally happy at the good news when I was confused by the other details. Still dwelling obsessively on the future, I became more emotionally fragile after the hospital visits than I had been for some time before. I was at odds with myself, and again started suffering from stress and anxiety. I was much better than immediately after the stroke, and I knew what I could not do in terms of returning to my previous life and lifestyle, yet I was overwhelmed by everything. The future only exists in our mind, and it was primarily the uncertainty that I feared.

In order to further establish why I may have had the stroke, I completed the 'Assessing your risk of stroke questionnaire', which has been established at the Mayo Clinic in Rochester, Minnesota. I answered each question honestly based on my lifestyle before the stroke. I did not even score high enough to get on the interpretation of results chart as a 'low risk' stroke candidate! Nevertheless, the exercise reinforced that illness is a great equaliser in life, and in terms of stroke, there is still a lot which is unknown. It was hard to continually try to pick myself up and get back on track. I don't believe there are any magical methods or tricks for doing this. I simply continued to organise my thoughts and tried to focus on the short term not the long term. I set myself a goal for the day and tried hard to achieve it with the 'players to the game' approach at the forefront of my mind (I explain more about this method in Chapter 10 'A Toolkit for Recovery and Prevention').

I knew very early on that I wanted to contribute to making a difference to other people affected by stroke. I soon joined the Stroke Association, and having read the accounts of other survivors I was finally able to tell people who asked how I was that I had had a stroke. I read the Association's information on depression after stroke and acknowledged that negative thinking and a loss of motivation could manifest themselves and cause further problems. As the months passed by, I started using imagery and chikung exercises more intensely (see Chapter 10). I saw myself doing what I wanted to do. I kept the images within realistic boundaries, but certainly ones that took me out of the comfort zone. As I went about each day, I kept affirming to myself that I had as many opportunities as I had ever had. To support this process, I dipped into a variety of self-help books and tried many different methods that are advocated for keeping positive.

I believe that during this time I started to develop a new rapport with myself, both physically and psychologically. I thought back to the words of my friend Andy: 'Right, you had better consider how you were pre-stroke is probably no longer the norm for you. Enjoy the memories and make the most of what the new norm might be.' It was obvious to me that I needed to have a good relationship with myself before I could really progress. The more choices I gave myself, the greater the chances of success. My beliefs and confidence would act as both permission for action and prohibition of achievement. I came to realise that I could actually decide how I wanted to feel. Anxiety is not something that is 'caught from someone else' (although negative people do not help!). My feelings of anxiety had been created as a result of the way in which I was viewing life due to the confusion and shock of surviving the stroke.

During this period of progress, which was made hard by the financial uncertainty of my future, I had a meeting with my friend and financial adviser Paul, who gave me an extract from a speech given by the former CEO of Coca-Cola Enterprises, Brian Dyson. As I read it for the first time, his comparison of life with the process of juggling balls in the air really struck a chord with me. Thinking of work as a rubber ball which, if dropped, will probably bounce, but thinking of family, friends and spirit as balls of glass which, if dropped, will at best be scuffed or at worst shattered, really helped me to put things into perspective. I have read the speech hundreds of times since being given it, and its value and worth to me is still as great now as the first time I read it.

Around this time a friend and teaching colleague of mine recommended a visit to a reflexologist (see Glossary) who he went to regularly. An inner ear problem meant that he would suddenly have to lie down in order to regulate his blood pressure and relieve feelings of nausea. This had been a problem for him for a few years, and for which his own doctors had not been able to regulate. He had even had to lie down in his classroom while teaching mathematics on occasions. The attacks seemed to happen regularly, every few weeks until he had reflexology, when they suddenly stopped. He had gone months without a recurrence when he recommended his reflexologist, Judith, to me. I made an appointment and was very impressed with Judith when I went for a consultation. I decided to continue using it as a way to help me to recover. Our approach was not to treat a specific problem, rather to encourage my body to rebalance its systems itself.

I also had a consultation with a 'life coach' (see Glossary). She was honest enough to tell me that in her opinion I was doing everything right in terms of looking to the future and would not benefit from working with her. I even attended a presentation given by an American mind and body expert. Although she had a distinct, trademarked system of self-development, I was pleased that essentially I had seemed to discover for myself what she and other people were advocating and practising.

Just a matter of weeks after my consultation with Dr Shetty at the University Hospital, I travelled back to the Royal Glamorgan Hospital for an outpatient appointment with a dietician. As I approached the hospital where I had been admitted I looked around at the people, and hustle and bustle. Were they visiting a friend or loved one? Were they celebrating good news like the birth of a grandchild or being admitted for major surgery? Had they just lost someone near and dear to them? Certainly, everyone seemed absorbed in their own world of thoughts and emotions. My appointment went well and the dietician confirmed that I had adapted my diet for the better. In addition, she confirmed that my triglyceride levels had also been tested and were perfectly normal.

In the weeks and months before I was able to face up to it, Anne decided to learn a little about stroke and what had happened to me. She read the booklets and discussed things with me. She was supportive, encouraging and respectful. She helped me to feel secure in my abilities to cope and helped me with confidence issues. Then again, Anne had always paid attention to the important things in a relationship.

I often received demonstrations of affection from her through looks, through being given small gifts, through hearing sensitive words, or just through being hugged. The whole experience has been understandably difficult for her, and even I have been surprised at times how strong she has been able to be for the most part. On one occasion, she came home from work, walked into the room where I was lying on the sofa and froze with the colour quickly draining from her cheeks. It transpired that her reaction was simply because I was wearing the T-shirt I had been wearing when I had suffered the stroke. Although it had been washed (several times), she explained that seeing me lying there wearing it gave her the immediate image of when she had first seen me in hospital some months earlier. That thought did not occur to me when I had put it on earlier in the day and I very quickly agreed to put it straight in the bin. However, on a second occasion, after having been out for no more than ten minutes, I returned home to find Anne crying. She had simply seen my slippers at the bottom of the stairs and started imagining that I might never have returned home from hospital to wear them again.

When trying to deal with a major life event such as stroke (including writing a book about it!), it is easy to become so self-absorbed that it is almost impossible to appreciate the insecurities developed by loved ones. Anne had obviously been deeply affected by my stroke and developed her own insecurities as a result. Having thought that I was going to die within hours of seeing me fit and strong has shaken her confidence greatly. To some extent, she has had to battle her own nerves and try to strike a balance between showing care and being overprotective. This is a fine line to walk and it took me many months to appreciate things from Anne's perspective!

However, as time went on, Anne would be less than impressed if she thought I was feeling sorry for myself. If I simply answered 'OK' when she would ask how I was, she would reply, 'Only OK?' She was right to point this out, no matter how trivial it may seem. If you wanted to buy the same model car as your friend, and he answered 'It's OK' when you asked 'How is it?', would you want to buy one? Probably not! 'OK' is not always acceptable, and we all want to feel, or be, better than it! My feeling is that by using positive language, including body language, at some level the brain believes this to be true and the mind will then try to act accordingly.

In short, Anne patiently supported me through this very emotional experience. For some time, I was losing my temper faster than I had ever done, and at times was even getting tired through the strain of trying to control it. My control over my emotions, which I had happily managed for almost 30 years, had been severely weakened, and maybe I was better for it. The feeling of anger that commonly follows a head injury tends to have a 'quick switch on' and a 'quick switch off'. I found that even when in a good mood it only took one small thing to irritate me and I would suddenly get very angry. My 'sensitised', or hypersensitive, state served to exaggerate all my emotions. Fortunately, the anger did not last because I was unable to concentrate on anything, even being angry, for long.

I was not really depressed, although clinical depression is common after suffering an adverse life event, such as a stroke. One school of thought is that depression may be some sort of survival mechanism by helping to conserve energy or by forcing withdrawal from situations that cause an individual to be anxious or under continuous risk. Indeed, doctors who treat depression believe that one of the most important steps to recovery is accepting it and not trying to fight it immediately. In this way, depression can be seen as a sign of strength and fighting, and should not have the common stigma of weakness, which is so readily associated with the condition. I wasn't particularly joyful at times, but I was coping. I think that my new-found emotional susceptibility helped me not to get depressed. The hormones released when I got angry seemed to be more powerful than any feelings I had when I was feeling slightly 'low'. While I was angry at the illness of stroke, my anger was often directed at Anne. Looking back, Anne came home from work some days not knowing what she would be faced with. Would I have the energy to open the door? Would I be happily preparing her evening meal in the kitchen with my new cook book open and wearing my new apron? Would I be in a stable, good mood, or would I be down and uncommunicative? Would I be anxious and nervous, or be feeling empowered and confident about the future? Would I manage to turn a friendly exchange into something more savage, causing her to end up in tears? Whatever she faced, she was consistent throughout. She greeted me with a loving smile. She asked how I was. She gave me a hug.

In my case, it was impossible to hold on to any feelings of anger for long. I am lucky in many ways. Anne is a natural performer and expert mimic with a razor-sharp wit. Occasionally she would insist on putting on a 'performance' in the house in an attempt to raise my spirits.

On one occasion when I was feeling a little low and had retreated to the bath to be on my own (something I rarely had time to do before the stroke), she waited until I was in it, and therefore a captive audience, and burst in performing a song-and-dance routine. Soon it turned into 'Stars in Their Eyes' as I had to act as the compere, tell her who to be and introduce her to

the audience, namely me in my bath. Another occasion saw her imperson-
ating Anne Robinson in her *Weakest Link* persona for virtually a whole evening. As the great entertainer Victor Borge is reported to have said,
'Laughter is the closest distance between two people.' I think that it is
highly likely that any chemicals released at these moments of pure laughter
were far greater than those causing me to feel 'low' or angry, and this phenomenon served me well. Michael Miller MD, director of the Center for
Preventative Cardiology at the University of Maryland Medical Center,
even suggests that the advice for a healthy heart may one day be a daily
combination of exercise, healthy eating and laughing (Murray 2004).

As well as entertaining me, Anne introduced essential oil burners
throughout the house and insisted on adding them to my bath. She introduced different oils in an attempt to provide either a calm and restful or
uplifting atmosphere in the house. Whether this worked or not, I am not
sure, but at least I always left the house smelling nice!

Despite my gratitude for all her care and attention, I nearly blew it on
one occasion. In March 2005, the Royal College of Physicians produced an
audit criticising the standard of stroke care in England and Wales. Following contact from the Stroke Association, I ended up giving an interview to a
newspaper about my experience. I was very nervous about doing it and
forgot to mention Anne at all. When I realised, I was just able to track down
and telephone the health editor to amend the article before it was submitted for print. Anne received her due credit, but it was a close call. The standard of care I had become used to might have taken a sudden turn for the
worse!

One thing I found during the months at home was that time had never
passed by so quickly. The hours turned quickly into days, the days into
weeks and very soon the weeks into months. I was never bored, and being
at home was certainly not the source of any mood swings. I would certainly
not have had any gender-role issues if Anne had become the sole breadwinner, and for a time we talked very seriously about whether that was a financially viable option. I had never felt defined as a person by what I did for a
living and would not have felt any less of a man if I did not work. I was
happy spending time as a 'househusband', and I even tried to make a chocolate mousse on one occasion. Unfortunately, I was still not as co-ordinated
as I would later become and spent a lot of my time cleaning much of it off
the toaster, window and kettle after trying to whisk it by hand.

While I was struggling with my own worries, one of our friends was
diagnosed with cancer, another lost a baby, and two of my former work colleagues died.

'See, it's not all about you!' Anne would say as we talked about life.

We shared in our friends' times of adversity and I came to realise that, to some extent, people were also sharing mine. I consciously made more time to appreciate what I had got, and I made the time to look forward, at least in the short term. My predominant emotion became one of a mixed state of calmness, as a result of my new daily routine, and happiness as to what the future might bring. I considered that before the stroke I was too busy with the daily routine of my life. Too busy basking in the ignorance that good health brings to enjoy looking forward to things. In so doing, I probably failed to appreciate experiences as much as I could have. If you have the time, looking forward to something certainly adds to the enjoyment.

Now, I am different. It may be that my increased appreciation for the small, but nevertheless important, things in life has made me more relaxed and actually strengthened my relationship with Anne. One of the really difficult things about experiencing a stroke is the fact that others around you want to help but inevitably will always be standing on the byline in some ways. It's also important to remember that strokes affect those around you, too. I tried, at times, to become a detached observer of what was happening to Anne and me after my stroke. I kept seeing her strength, love, honesty and humour holding us together. This made my attempts to remain positive more purposeful and probably more enjoyable. Anne was concerned throughout our time 'post-stroke' about any personality changes in me, and after several months she admitted that I had changed. She thought that I had developed a sense of humour! On reflection, I can think of easier ways to have done this.

Dogs and more therapy

Several months after signing up, we had our first guide dog to stay. He was a wonderful black Labrador called Woody. Woody arrived with the usual equipment, including a guide dog lead, and took me by surprise the first time we took him out to the park. Anne and I thought that a walk around the park's lake with all the ducks, swans and rowing boats would make for a pleasant afternoon. It was a sunny summer's day and I was wearing sunglasses while walking with Woody, who was on his lead, not realising what it looked like to other walkers. Unfortunately, we did not realise that this would be the first time for Woody to see a duck. He gave chase towards the lake, taking me with him. My balance was still poor at this time, as was my strength, and before Anne knew what was happening I was several metres away. I was somehow able to keep up with Woody until I hit the first tree, which I managed to keep hold of. As Anne stood laughing, Woody spotted bread a short distance to his right that had obviously been left for the ducks. With this, he realised that I had no control over him and dragged me over to the bread, which he ate like a wild boar. I shouted to Anne, 'I can't do it!' It was at that moment, as she made her way over to us, that I realised I had the sympathy of the other walkers, many with young children, who obviously thought that I was blind and had a rogue dog!

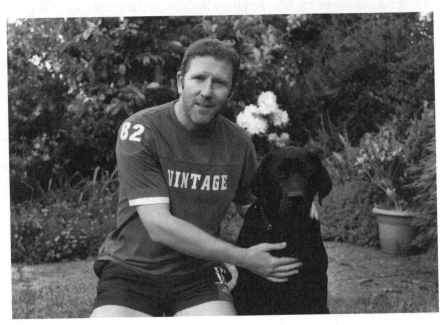

Me with Woody

A few months later we looked after a real character, a golden retriever called Floyd, who had been given early retirement on 'disciplinary grounds'. As a result he was with us for seven months, which was a great motivation for me to leave the house and continue to walk every day. Despite being with us such a long time his stay went smoothly – apart from when he found a sex toy in a bush and tried to trot around the park with it in his mouth. I certainly didn't want to try to take it off him in case he thought it was a game of tug-of-war. In the end he gave it to me. When I told Anne she didn't believe me – until I produced the item as proof!

Just before Floyd arrived, Dr Shetty told me that I could start swimming. This was a real struggle at first. I battled to lift my left arm out of the water and my legs felt heavy and dragged low. I could not swim in a straight line, and had to utilise floats in order to improve. Despite briefly feeling down at the fact I could not swim as I had done before (I held many school records as a junior and was a qualified lifeguard as an adult) I was inspired to persevere by the other swimmers around me, many of whom were over 70 years old and swam past me with ease. So I set about improving my strength and muscle tone by applying the 'principles of training' that are described in Chapter 10, and I added a morning swim to my daily routine. This was hard physically, but it was only due to the commitment I made to myself that I maintained this in the cold winter months, and when I was in no mood to go.

My swimming sessions, especially with an imbalance between each side of my body and certain muscles compensating for others, led to some more aches and discomfort. My lower back and left shoulder in particular caused problems. A close friend who is a sports massage therapist, Paul, suggested that he could help. With Dr Shetty's permission, on the understanding that my neck was to be avoided, he set to work on me. With the exception of my neck, which Dr Shetty stipulated should not receive attention due to the VAD, Paul worked on my shoulders, back, pelvic girdle and legs. Details of sports massage therapy (SMT) are provided in Chapter 10, but I would say here and now, the results were miraculous. However, the massage techniques are deep and certainly not for the faint-hearted. I only lasted ten minutes at our first session before I had to tell Paul to stop, as I felt sick. Again, and with Paul's patience, I persevered and our session became a fortnightly event with each treatment lasting 45 minutes. As far as my physical progress is concerned, SMT with Paul is undoubtedly one of the most useful 'players to the game' that I incorporated into my routine.

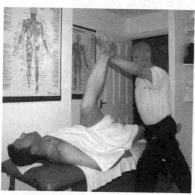
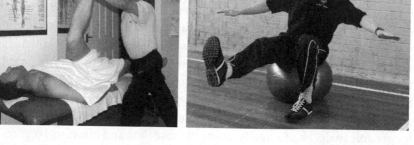

Massage therapy with Paul   *Me working on developing some core strength*

Two months into the massage therapy, Steve Cannon, a chartered physio-therapist who had treated me for sports injuries over many years, heard that I had had the stroke and got in touch. He had worked a lot with stroke patients before opening his private practice in Cardiff and very kindly offered his services. Despite my knowledge of anatomy, physiology and how the body works, and therefore of the benefits of good physiotherapy, I had not initiated contact with Steve. This was due to a mixture of not accepting the effects of the stroke, some ignorance as to how he could actu-ally help, and the fact that he knew me so well before the stroke. However, working with him took my physical recovery to another level, helping develop my core strength: the muscles around the waist and back which are pivotal to all movement and stability. As uncomfortable as it was, I worked for many hours on the exercises he set me, and was even able to incorporate them and do them while typing at my desk. I thought back to the famous words of Winston Churchill and applied them to my situation, 'If you're going through hell, keep going!' More detail of these exercises is described in Chapter 10.

Before long, the anniversary of my stroke arrived. It was a strange day. I am not good with dates and have always failed to remember friends' birth-days and wedding anniversaries. However, the date of my stroke never leaves my mind. This is also true for Anne and my parents. Anne bought me a present to mark the ocassion, and my mother was also quite excited that the date came and went, this time with me 'behaving myself with no antics' (Anne's words!). Since then, I have noticed that many stroke survivors refer to the exact date, and even the time, of their stroke when talking about their experience.

With this day having passed, I gradually came to feel very comfortable with the new pace I had set myself. However, these feelings were short-lived – that same month I received some quite disappointing news. I was unable to return to my teaching job, a fact recognised by the Teachers Pen-sions Department, and had applied for ill health retirement from teaching a month earlier. Much to everyone's surprise, my application was initially denied. I am led to believe that this would largely have been as a result of my age. This served as an example of how the illness of stroke is still misun-derstood and vague even in the eyes of medical examiners. Is it not possible that something could be even more devastating age 37 than 77? Still, ques-tions like that are largely academic, and the plain truth was that I had con-scientiously devoted virtually my whole adult life to a job that I was no longer able to do. I had actually devoted more time and effort to 16 years of work than many people do in 40 years. With the support of my union, colleagues and doctors an appeal was submitted against the original decision, and it was actually a further nine months before this matter was resolved and I was granted ill health retirement as a result of the stroke. The detrimental impact of this whole affair on my confidence and attitude, let alone my thoughts and plans for the future, cannot be overstated, and things were difficult for a time while I tried to work through my thoughts again.

Around this time I paid for a few private sessions with a consultant psychiatrist, having already attended counselling sessions as arranged by my GP. Initially, I suppose, I was sceptical about how I would benefit, but the sessions confirmed to me that the anxiety I suffered concerned the uncertainty about my teaching post and adjusting to such a major life event. It was pointed out to me that I still retained many of the positive character traits I had before the stroke, and in our consultations we identified that the psychological trauma associated with stroke is often overlooked by physicians, and widely misunderstood by society. We highlighted that the recovery and rehabilitation work that I had been doing was very much in keeping with how I had lived my life before the stroke. Specifically, that I was engrossed in improving physical performance. Inevitably, I had not fully addressed all the psychological issues. Eventually, we employed strategies for reducing anxiety and agreed that I should explore any opportunities to work for myself.

'Opportunity is missed by most people because it is dressed in overalls and looks like work.'

Thomas Edison (1847–1931)

~ Chapter 5 ~

Walking a New Path

With the exception of my brain, most of my body had changed from the one that had had the stroke. The cells of the eyes replace themselves in three days; the stomach lining is replaced in less than a week; the skin cells do the same over a period of four weeks; the skeleton every three months; and the liver every six months. In addition, my perspectives had also changed. I made more time to talk to myself and re-establish the very important rapport with the world around me and, equally importantly, the rapport with myself. Unfortunately, developing rapport with self seems to be something that is often overlooked in today's society.

I came to know myself better, as a direct result of my experience, and found a sensitivity that had been hidden for years. I had hoped to avoid the crying associated with stroke survivors, but cracked after nine months. My emotions suddenly took me and Anne (and Floyd!) completely by surprise when I began to have bouts of (very loud) crying. However, I reconciled myself with my newly developed personality, and accepted that these new feelings may pop out from time to time.

I continued reading a range of self-help books, because no matter how much I thought about it, and I did think about it every day, I was at a complete loss in terms of the direction I wanted my life to go in. I was pleased to read that many of the tools and the mindset advocated in such books were already firmly ingrained in my approach and 'toolkit for recovery' (Chapter 10). So I decided to become my own life coach and simply approached it as if I was advising a loved one. I had spent many years as a sports coach and teacher reaffirming the achievements of others. I know that some of my students achieved success simply because they knew that I believed in them. Therefore, I actively invested time in developing the habit of thinking positively, which in turn helped me to understand more about the process of recovery after a major life event like a stroke. I have no doubt that this helped to trigger responses in my unconscious mind, which in turn helped to strengthen my resolve to move forward.

The recovery process .

- Moving through phases of shock, denial, anger and acceptance
- Reduction in swelling to the stroke-affected area of the brain
- Medical intervention as appropriate
- Rest to aid natural recovery
- Natural re-routing of neurological pathways in the brain
- Occupational, physiological and complementary therapy
- Adaptation of lifestyle to aid the coping experience (as required)
- Stroke survivor's willingness to persevere
- Remembering that the recovery process does not stop

I also praised myself for the many hours of physical therapy I undertook on my own. I thought back to how, as a teacher, I was encouraged to offer praise and to celebrate the achievements of those I taught; and I thought how, in our society, it is more difficult to celebrate the 'small' achievements of adults. Celebration is a good thing. It evokes an emotional response and triggers an emotional memory. With time, I reconnected with the positive memories and self-belief I had before the stroke. I reaffirmed my goals for the future. I used a variety of tools to help with this. These tools ranged from positive self-talk by saying out loud to myself 'I am genuinely happy and moving forward' to writing down my goals and reading them every day. I used to have to learn for exams by repeatedly writing down what I had learnt. The physical act of writing the goals gave me a clear vision, which I believe extended from my conscious deep into my subconscious and in so doing programmed my brain to seek out ways to fulfil the goals. I always performed well under examination conditions as a result, and could see no reason why this technique should be any less effective in the context of goal-setting. Writing a goal is a dynamic technique, which starts the process of action and reinforces the goal at a subconscious level. Before long, I had a diverse, challenging and fairly extensive list of goals. Some I have now achieved. Some I achieve on a daily basis. Others I am continually working towards. As I work towards these goals, I often remember one of my favourite pieces of teaching advice: 'Don't measure yourself by what you have accomplished, but by what you should have accomplished with your abilities' (attributed to US college basketball coach John Wooden).

For a stroke survivor, as with anyone else, there are many methods available to help establish goals. However, a stroke survivor may feel at more of a crossroads than other individuals. It may be that an element of reframing is needed to confirm the significance of choices that have already been made or, having survived a stroke, it's not too strong a term to say that, for some, the aim may actually move from goal-setting and extend to identifying life's purpose. Based on his experience of battling cancer, Robin Sieger came to the conclusion that we are able to design our lives from the end back. He believes that we should think of the things we would like to have said about us at the end of our life, and what we want to have achieved. As a useful exercise, we could even write a personal obituary that we would be proud of and set about making it happen. This is probably based on the story about Alfred Nobel, a 19th-century Swedish armaments manufacturer. It is reported that on opening a newspaper one day, he was most surprised to read a headline claiming that he had just died. He quickly realised that the paper must have made an identity mistake, as it was his brother, Ludvig, who had just died. As he read the article fully, he was disturbed to find that the obituary was indeed his own. Alfred Nobel had made a fortune after discovering and patenting dynamite and expected to read a very complimentary article. Instead, he realised that people saw him as a 'merchant of death', making his money on the back of war. On reading his obituary, he discovered his true life's purpose and immediately set new goals and devoted himself, and his wealth, to science, the arts and peace. The result, the Nobel Prize, is now the world's most respected award.

Another useful method of identifying a purpose in life, or equally importantly some simple goals, starts with imagining that it's some time in the future: the choice of timeframe can be entirely personal. The task then is to write a self-addressed postcard, which identifies what you are doing, what you enjoy about your life and mentioning how you got there. Again such a simple yet positive action helps in realising that goals are achievable.

Both of these methods, along with many others that are available, cut through many peripheral issues and take a person towards their 'being self' rather than their 'doing self'. Should you choose to use any of them, be prepared – the goal or purpose you identify may come as a bit of a shock!

One of the interesting and pertinent books I read about goal-setting was *Did You Spot the Gorilla? How to Recognise Hidden Opportunities* (Wiseman 2004). It is based on the premise that the world is now a faster and more pressured place than ever before, but that we are all primed and encouraged to think, conform and behave in the same way as always. The result is that we have 'psychological blindspots' causing us to miss a great deal of opportunities in our lives, many of which are obvious. The book's title is based on a study using a 30-second film made by Harvard psychologist Daniel Simons. To put it briefly, he directed an audience to count the passes made by a team in a basketball match. By following these instructions, and behaving in the way expected of them, very few of the audience spotted a man dressed in a gorilla costume who walks through the basketball players and beats his chest. This remains a common phenomenom with those who watch this film under Simons's experimental conditions. Therefore, the 'gorilla' in Wiseman's book is simply a metaphor for the 'blindspots' that cause us to miss simple solutions and opportunities, which could transform our lives.

To help me spot 'gorillas' in the future, I began to (and continue to) use a range of tools, including some suggested by Wiseman. I hope that my experience of stroke will encourage me to spot 'gorillas' and to see the bigger picture within my life. In very simplistic terms, I have been influenced by stroke in much the same way as I am influenced by fashion (although according to Anne, I am not influenced by fashion at all!). I would not wear the clothes of 15 years ago, and now I do not have the same goals of 15 years ago. My new 'norm' and new goals combine the delicate mix of the physical and psychological pieces that I have reassembled post-stroke in order to continue to live what I hope will be a most rewarding life.

I no longer feel the need to compete with others in the way that I did before the stroke, but still very much like to compete with myself. I know that ingrained somewhere in the philosophy of competition is the desire for celebration. The scale of the celebration will obviously vary, depending either on the profile of the competition or on the personality of the individual. I have always known that I have been a little too 'British', in that I have been embarrassed to celebrate much of my successes through life. I suppose, with hindsight, most of the time I have been too busy to take the time to recognise, celebrate and reflect. Now, celebration has almost become a habit as I try to recognise and celebrate something every day – even if it is just the simple act of reflecting on the simple things in life. When I was lying in hospital in the early hours and days after the stroke and was worrying about what I might have lost, the quality of my car, our TV and audio equipment or the money in my bank account just did not enter my head. Instead, I worried about the simple things. I worried about my daily routine, the things that I had previously taken very much for granted and the people who contribute to making my life what it is. These are the things that I valued and these are the things that I now take time out every day to celebrate.

It is very easy to become complacent, and so I try to remember that time is passing by and no day will ever come again.

I have no doubt that the act of consciously appreciating the simple things led to me regaining some of the confidence I had had before the stroke. This in turn resulted in me stepping out of the comfort zone and wanting to learn new skills again. I started with driving, and enrolled on the Institute of Advanced Motorists advanced driving course, which I was pleased to pass first time.

Some time later, I enrolled on an excellent Clinical Hypnotherapy Practitioner Diploma course with the Brief Strategic Therapy (BST) Foundation in London. This was demanding, stimulating and was of real use to me in helping to understand the power of the mind a little better. In addition, the skills I learnt are ones that I anticipate being of real value to me, and others, in the future. One of the simplest techniques I learnt allowed me to give a short speech to my former teaching colleagues when I was invited back to school and was given a very generous leaving gift by the Staff Association. To be honest I tried to get out of it knowing that I would be under a bit of pressure to say a few words, but as the day approached I practised my speech for a couple of hours and used a simple anatomical triggering technique to keep calm and apply feelings of confidence to the moment. In the end my speech was delivered perfectly without the need for notes. The result was that a fear of speaking to an audience which I had developed after the stroke, and what I perceived as an awkward situation, was overcome successfully. I had always been happy talking to very large and sometimes very demanding audiences, and laughed at the fact that people often say they would rather be dead than speak in public. At least now I have developed an understanding of why people feel this way.

As time went on and I started to think more clearly about the future, I attended a very good business course run by Business in Focus in Wales, specifically for people who are interested in working for themselves.

As my confidence grew, and as part of my goal-setting therapy, I visualised and made myself believe that my series of notes would make it into print. In fact, this was one of the goals that I wrote down. I wanted to contribute to:

• raising awareness of issues relating to stroke

• understanding how strokes can be prevented

- informing society about how strokes affect individuals

- raising awareness of the burden that strokes place on society

- providing information about some of the practices that can assist recovery in stroke survivors.

It seemed to me that as strokes can kill or severely disable, many of those most deeply affected are unable to help with the education of others. Unlike many who survive heart attacks or cancer, stroke survivors are often only able to live in relative isolation from the outside world. I hoped that my experiences and the road I took to recovery would, in some small way, register with and help others affected by stroke. After all, opportunities pass, they don't pause. I have now learnt not to define myself simply as someone who has had a stroke. In the same way, I am also not defined by the car that I drive or the jobs I have done. Nor do I perceive myself as an *ex*

How to move on

- Dare to dream – rediscover the excitement of having dreams for the future.

- Concentrate on strengths not weaknesses – this is not a corrective process.

- Be aware of your own excuses.

- Integrate action on a daily basis – set, acknowledge and share goals.

- Develop affirmations – use positive, present tense statements.

- Think that the goal has already been achieved – if possible, also act as if the goal has already been achieved.

- Accept infallibility and life's ebbs and flow – don't give up during a 'plateau'.

- Celebrate small success – this validates your investment in time and action.

- Celebrate personal triumphs.

- Create a timeline from a place in the future – this creates that 'thrill of a chase'.

- Look out for 'gorillas'!

anything just because I no longer do it. Nor do I perceive myself as a swimmer just because I regularly go to a pool to work out. I no longer consider myself to be defined by any labels such as these. I now accept, perhaps for the first time, that I am much more than the sum total of such things.

I have thought long and hard about whether I would be where I am now, in terms of my personal development, if I had not had the stroke. I have come to the conclusion that I would not. As I used to say when teaching martial art seminars, 'If you do what you've always done, you'll get what you've always got.' I have been forced to change what I've always done and am now able to reflect on the fact that I have seen into the world of stroke with my own eyes. I have survived. I feel liberated by the experience and now, as I am walking a new path, I am spotting 'gorillas' everywhere!

Part II

An Introduction to Neuroscience: A Route Through the Maze of Information

As a direct result of my own first-hand experience of stroke, and my educational background, which includes the study of anatomy and physiology and health, the following chapters will, I hope, provide some clarity of the main physiological issues of stroke. I think that the simplest way to do this is by considering the following:

- What is a stroke? (Chapter 6)

- What do we know about the brain and its blood supply? (Chapter 7)

- What happens before and during a stroke, and why? (Chapter 8)

- What are the short- and long-term effects of stroke? (Chapter 9)

I must point out that I write this as someone with no medical training, and I write this for someone with no medical training to be able to read and understand. I am sure you would agree that we would all benefit from a basic understanding of the human body, even if it just makes it easier to communicate with the medical profession. There are over one thousand disorders of the brain and nervous system, and so any information that helps to improve our understanding of this aspect of organic function may prove useful. For those of you reading this who are stroke patients or stroke patient relatives, it may be that this part of the book will assist you to become better diagnostic and/or treatment partners with your doctors, therapists and carers. I hope, therefore, that you will find here a suitable, understandable amount of relevant information, which can be considered in the context of stroke.

Chapter 6

What Is a Stroke?

A stroke, as you will have gathered throughout this book, is serious – just like a heart attack. The term 'stroke' is used to describe the neurological damage caused by an abnormal blood flow to the brain. Please understand and have no doubt that a stroke, sometimes now called a 'cerebrovascular accident' or 'brain attack' (see Glossary), is most definitely a medical emergency.

The term 'brain attack' in relation to stroke is credited to Vladimir C. Hachinski and John Norris, both world-renowned neurologists from Canada. It has become more widely used in recent years because it characterises the medical condition and communicates to the public the actual event more clearly than the word 'stroke'. The doctors and organisations that advocate the use of the term 'brain attack' believe that the general misperception that nothing can be done about stroke has prevailed for too long. By using the term 'brain attack', they give stroke a definitive name and a unique profile. Of all the images used to identify stroke, brain attack is possibly the most descriptive, providing an immediate image and immediate connotation.

The medical concept of stroke has been in existence for over 2000 years, but it has only been since the 17th century that the causes of stroke have begun to be understood. In the event of a stroke, the symptoms occur in the body but the stroke actually occurs in the brain. You need to understand that in our body, the blood carries oxygen and nutrients to the brain, and takes away carbon dioxide and cellular waste. As a stroke generally happens when normal blood flow to the brain stops, the brain does not then receive the amount of glucose and oxygen it needs and brain cells begin to die.

The most common category of stroke is that caused by a blood clot that blocks a blood vessel or artery in the brain. This has been likened to when a city is under siege and starvation is the result (Wiebers 2001). In this simple analogy, people die in a city under siege when food is no longer supplied;

and in the case of stroke, brain cells die in the brain when blood is not supplied. This type of stroke is called an ischaemic stroke.

The second, and least common, category of stroke is a haemorrhagic stroke. This is caused when a blood vessel in the brain ruptures (the main reasons for this are given later), spilling blood into the surrounding tissue. Dr Wiebers again explains this effectively with a second analogy. He likens a haemorrhage to flood damage. Flooding, when caused by a leakage or breaking of a dam, can be catastrophic, damaging or displacing all in its path. In the case of stroke a flood of blood occurs in the brain and puts pressure on brain tissue, affecting its function and sometimes causing the surrounding arteries to spasm (which may in turn result in ischaemic stroke).

Both ischaemic and haemorrhagic strokes clearly cause damage to the brain, but in very different ways. Either way, brain cells in the area affected begin to die (this will be further developed later). The symptoms of each type of stroke may or may not be different (on this note, I think that is worth reminding you again that whatever the cause, some people recover completely from stroke, while other individuals lose their lives to stroke), but they require very different medical treatment.

Ischaemic strokes

As mentioned above, a stroke caused by a blood clot is referred to as an 'ischaemic stroke'. Ischaemia is a lack of blood flow to an organ, whereas 'hyponoxia' or 'anoxia' (other common terms) is the interrupted oxygen supply to the brain. The area of the brain damaged by the loss of oxygen is called the 'infarct'.

It may be helpful to know that the medical profession classify ischaemic strokes by their cause. Ischaemic strokes originate, for the most part, outside of the brain. In some cases, there may have been a problem within the blood itself (e.g. sickle cell disease); there may exist a blood vessel disorder (e.g. arteritis); or the stroke may have occurred as the result of a build-up of atherosclerotic plaque which reduced blood flow to the brain. However, most ischaemic strokes are caused by a blood clot. The blood clot and any subsequent stroke is then often categorised again as either:

- a thrombus and a thrombotic stroke (when the clot blocks a vessel that supplies an area of the brain with blood)

or:

- an embolus and an embolic stroke (when the clot originates elsewhere in the body and travels to the brain, becoming wedged in a vessel that supplies the brain with blood).

Both a thrombus and embolus are among the aspects shown in Figure 8.1, should you find it useful to look ahead to page 141.

Haemorrhagic strokes

A haemorrhagic stroke is a stroke caused by a bleed. Haemorrhagic strokes originate within the brain itself and, unlike ischaemic strokes, are categorised in terms of the location of the haemorrhage. In such cases, the cause of bleeding can include a blow to the head; the rupture of a blood vessel within the brain, which may have been weakened by years of hypertension; the use of recreational drugs; or an aneurysm or malformation. The latter is illustrated in Figure 7.6, should you find it useful to look ahead to page 135.

While there are five types of brain haemorrhage, not all are considered to be types of stroke. Generally, those caused through a head injury are unlikely to be included in stroke statistics. However, the following two categories are considered as stroke:

- a subarachnoid haemorrhage, which accounts for between 5 and 10 per cent of all strokes (in the UK this equates to around 8500 cases per year), with women being the most likely to experience one – the bleed occurs within the space between the brain and the skull, known as the arachnoid space, and just 10cc of escaping blood is enough to be disastrous

- an intracerebral haemorrhage, which accounts for between 10 and 15 per cent of all strokes and occurs within the brain itself; while the cause can be any of those stated above for a haemorrhagic stroke, the most common cause of an intracerebral haemorrhage is hypertension.

I think that it is worth remembering, as it will be of further help and guidance when we later examine the effects of stroke, that ischaemic strokes are generally (although there are exceptions) unilateral in nature affecting just one hemisphere of the brain, but the bleeding of a haemorrhagic stroke may affect both hemispheres of the brain, depending on its size and location. It is also worth bearing in mind that there are other conditions with symptoms similar to stroke which can make early diagnosis difficult. These include abnormal blood chemistry (e.g. low sodium levels), abnormal arterio-venous blood vessels, alcohol or drug intoxication, a brain abscess or tumour, epilepsy and a range of psychological problems.

Chapter 7

The Brain and Its Blood Supply

Basic neuro-anatomy for the lay person

In order to further understand the illness of stroke, and before we attempt to interpret the various symptoms, and appreciate the many effects, I believe that it is first necessary to know some basic neuro-anatomy in relation to the brain. Even the most fundamental information provides interesting reading, and I certainly benefited, in trying to learn more about stroke, from having an understanding of what a healthy brain is made of and what it actually does. That said, there is still a great deal for scientists and doctors to learn about the brain, and even in the 21st century there is more that is not known than there is known about this most complex of organs.

I embarked upon a fascinating journey of discovery about the brain when researching this book. From teaching anatomy and physiology, I had a basic understanding of its role, but on reflection was still incredibly naïve as to what it actually does. I make no claims to be medically competent on issues relating to the brain, but I know that if you remember that the brain is like a boardroom of experts existing primarily to support the body, you will better understand the information contained in this chapter. While you may never have attempted to familiarise yourself with any aspect of anatomy or physiology before, remember, the average person undoubtedly invests more time in establishing how their CD player, VCR, DVD player or PC works, than they do in acquiring the same amount of information about how their brain works. It will be worth spending some time reading this chapter.

The brain and its interaction with the nervous system

Our brain really sets us apart from all other species. It is a collection of differentiated but homogeneous (the same kind of) structures. However, no two brains are identical and even identical twins have visible differences in brain structure at birth. Our brains, like our faces, all contain the same

Brain facts

- The brain and spinal cord make up the central nervous system.
- The central nervous system controls everything that the human body and mind does.
- The human brain weighs around 1200g.
- The brain accounts for approximately 2 per cent of our body weight.
- The brain consumes 20 per cent of the oxygen produced by the cardio-vascular system.
- Neurones are the cells that create brain activity.
- Each individual cell or neurone is in contact with up to 2000 other nerve cells.
- The brain itself can be injured by trauma, disease and stroke.

regions but are not identical to one another. In each of us, some regions are specialised while others have a more general purpose. However, there are common features that can be considered:

- the brain is largely protected from external physical trauma by the skull
- the brain is largely protected from internal biological damage by membranes and fluid
- the brain is a jelly-like substance that contains over 1000 trillion connections of 100 billion nerve cells
- it generates more electrical impulses in a day than the combined total of all the world's telephones.

Each nerve cell in the brain is referred to as a neurone, and neurones are the largest cells in the body. There are different types, but they are able to connect to other neurones through extensions out of them (called axons) and projections from them (called dendrites). These connections, as evident in Figure 7.1, carry an electrical signal from one neurone to another and form a two-way system. The axons, also called the nerve fibre, send out signals and the dendrites receive signals. Both the spinal cord and the brain consist of white matter (bundles of axons) and grey matter (high density mass of neurones and dendrites). In the brain, the grey matter is not continuous but is seen in various collections, or nuclei, of grey matter.

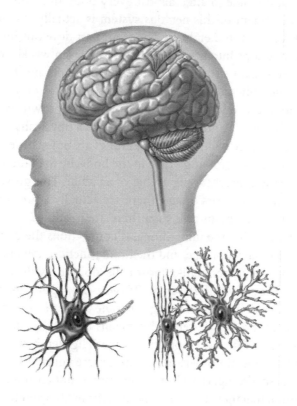

Figure 7.1: Side view of the brain showing the outer brain structure, and nerve cells. Illustration by Philip Wilson FMAA RMIP. Reproduced with permission from the Brain and Spine Foundation.

All sensation, movements, thoughts, memories and feelings are the result of signals that pass through these neurones. When the signal is received, it stimulates the release of a chemical neurotransmitter. The effect of the neurotransmitter can sometimes be 'excitatory', in that it influences other systems, or it can be 'inhibitory', which is when it does not influence other systems because it would cause an unwanted effect. Examples of neurotransmitters relevant to strokes include acetylcholine (for muscle control) and endorphin (for disrupting signals from pain receptors).

These complex communication pathways allow parts of the brain to be informed about what is happening in other parts, and in a healthy person, the speed of nerve conduction can reach a staggering 220 miles per hour. A single neurone can receive and process information from up to 100,000 other neurones. As a result, the brain never switches off and is constantly monitoring, and is able to alter, almost every body function.

The development of this nervous system is actually visible along the back of a three-week-old embryo. The front part develops into the brain, and the rest develops into the spinal cord. Just seven weeks after conception, the brain's main structures (forebrain, midbrain and hindbrain) are visible. Unbelievably, in a developing foetus a quarter of a million brain cells are produced every minute. The result of this growth is that a new-born child has the same number of neurones as a physically mature adult, the obvious difference being that the neurones are not mature. However, as the brain is the fastest-growing organ in the body, by the time a child is two years old its brain is nearly as big as that of an adult. This growth is unique to humans, and at six years of age, there are actually a greater number of connections between brain cells than there are in adults.

As we grow older, the unused neural connections die back, the brain suffers some natural shrinkage, and the brain functions become quite rigid and distinctive. Neurones, unlike most cells, do not divide and reproduce and are irreplaceable. In the average 75-year-old, approximately 50,000 neurones a day will have been dying for some 50 years, resulting in a total depletion of around 10 per cent. This means that at this stage in life, the brain is receiving a fifth less blood and is a tenth lighter than it was aged 20. However, the connections between neurones are constantly evolving and being refined, so a comparable loss of function is not an automatic result. I should mention that there may be some specific mental abilities and gender differences in brain performance as a result of the ageing process, but I will not go into detail about this here.

The brain itself is responsible for maintaining and regulating all basic body functions; intelligence, learning and memory; moral and social behaviour; the interpretation of sensory information (sight, hearing, smell, taste and touch); and initiating and controlling all purposeful body movements, balance and co-ordination.

In other words, it does everything and is the control centre of our nervous system, the interconnected parts of which are illustrated in Figure 7.2. So, as illustrated, even when we are asleep, the brain is constantly receiving and interpreting information from every part of the body. With such complexity, perhaps it should be more of a wonder that so many brains operate so well, and for so long!

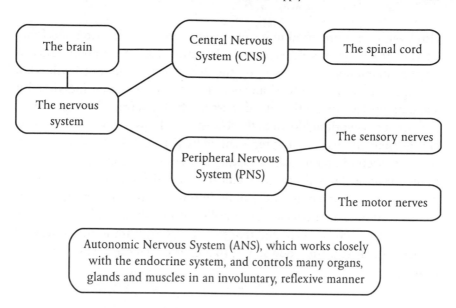

Figure 7.2: The interconnected parts of the nervous system

The brain and its sections

Any study of the brain must involve dividing it into sections or mapping it according to function. Initially, mapping it according to function was dependent on the study of patients with localised damage and some associated and specific deficits. As a result, stroke patients were among the earliest subjects, and the language areas of the brain were among the first to be thoroughly studied. While much more is known now than even in recent history, the study of brain function and the independence of the component sub-functions is still very much ongoing, via many scientific and academic disciplines. As a result, many anatomists, biologists, neurologists and neuropsychologists present the subgroups or map of the brain in different ways for teaching purposes, the presentation of theory and for information purposes. For example, some present information in a chronological way based on the evolution of the brain (from the oldest parts to the newest), and others divide it from front to back. For these purposes, the brain might be divided into three and any of the following terminology may be used:

- forebrain (also known as the prosencephalon)
- midbrain (mesencephalon)
- hindbrain (rhombencephalon).

However, I have preferred to develop and present the location and functions of the brain in a different way. The information I present below is quite a common way of presenting the different sections, but I will work through it in a 'nose to toes' manner. In other words, if an individual is standing up, I am presenting and discussing the brain from the highest part and gradually working down to the lowest part. How I view and will present the brain in this section is represented by Figure 7.3. I think that this is the most useful in terms of developing a three-dimensional picture of the brain for those of us who are not medically trained, but who simply wish to develop an understanding of the brain in relation to stroke. While I make some mention about how blood is supplied as I work through each section (you will have already gathered that this is very relevant in the context of stroke), I do discuss the blood supply to the brain in more detail later in this chapter.

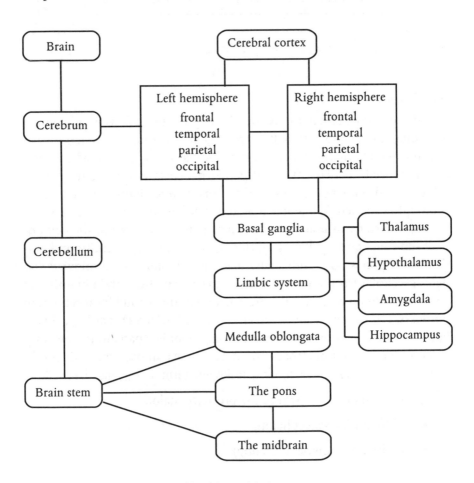

Figure 7.3: A basic neuro-anatomical breakdown of the brain

The evolution of the human brain and nervous system is actually reflected in its structure. The brain and nervous system evolved upwards and outwards by adding on to what was already there. Simply speaking, the oldest parts deal with reflexes while the newer layers are associated with memory, learning and thinking.

Deep inside the brain is the limbic system. This is the primitive, unconscious area of the brain, which governs self-preservation. The next largest portion of the brain is the cerebellum, which is followed in size by the brainstem. These sections both regulate a wide range of bodily functions and movement. The most recently evolved area of the brain is the cerebral cortex, which is responsible for all the brain's higher mental functions (such as language processing). The cerebral cortex covers the largest portion of the brain, the cerebrum. The cerebral cortex and cerebrum are split geographically into a number of lobes. These are the frontal, temporal, parietal and occipital lobes, which are actually named after the skull bones that lie directly over them. Again, you may find it beneficial to look ahead to Figure 8.1 as the lobes are identified very clearly.

In the same way that the human brain evolved from the deepest and most primitive sections, the process of mental maturation of the human brain also starts in these sections. For example, young babies display simple emotional reactions associated with instinct and mood as a result of the activity within the limbic system. Soon, they are able to make simple decisions, understand language, and eventually speak. Again, similar to how the human brain evolved, the working development of each individual human brain as it passes through puberty and into adulthood is also upwards and outwards.

The cerebral cortex

The cerebral cortex is a thin layer of nerve cell bodies that covers the outer surface of the cerebrum. The cerebral cortex is also known as the grey matter, a term often associated with intelligence. It is found under three layers of protective tissue known as the 'meninges'. One of these layers, the 'dura mater', is labelled in Figure 7.6. Beneath the cerebral cortex lies the cerebrum, or white matter.

The cerebrum

The cerebrum is the largest part of the brain, accounting for a fifth of its weight, and controls voluntary actions, thought, speech and memory. It 'defines us as humans' (Hachinski and Hachinski 2004). Due to the process of evolution, it is sometimes called the 'mammalian' brain. Most mammals actually have a relatively small cerebrum, but in humans it makes up most of the brain and evolved around 160 million years ago. It is divided into two halves, called the left and right hemispheres (evident in Figure 7.4).

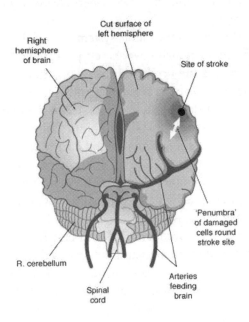

Figure 7.4: View of a brain showing stroke damage and the surrounding penumbral region that is at risk of damage. Illustration reproduced with kind permission from Professor Richard Morris and the British Neuroscience Association.

At birth, each hemisphere has the potential to perform every mental skill on its own. It is possible that a child could lose an entire hemisphere and still develop quite normally with the remaining hemisphere doing all the work. That said, minor differences between the hemispheres do make each one best suited to certain tasks. Without doubt, as a result of the ageing process, these minor differences and the subsequent use and development of each hemisphere become entrenched in how each one operates. Therefore, the loss of function of a hemisphere in later life, through injury such as stroke, can have catastrophic consequences.

As the brain develops from infancy through to adulthood, the hemispheres are said to act unilaterally with regard to some functions. For example, the left hemisphere largely controls the right side of the body, whereas the right side of the brain controls the left side. The left side solves problems using logic. The right cerebral hemisphere controls our feelings, thoughts and creative inclinations. The advertising world recognises this and spends millions of pounds exploiting the vulnerability of the right hemisphere by showing us visual images rather than supplying us with logical messages that are more likely to be rejected by the left hemisphere. A good advert is simply one that encourages us to act on impulse by making us think that we are acting as the result of a logical decision.

The left hemisphere seems to be the 'optimistic' half of the brain, and perhaps offers some control over all our emotions. It is associated with positive emotions (e.g. happiness, joy and pleasure). The right side is the 'pessimistic' half and is often associated with negative emotions (e.g. anger, sorrow and general feelings of being moody and bad-tempered).

In left-handed individuals there is perhaps less of a disproportionate dominance between the two hemispheres – activity is spread more evenly between the two halves of the brain. Perhaps this is why left-handed people are considered to be more artistic, or more emotional, while right-handed people seem to be more thoughtful, less emotional, even more clinical. An extreme example of this can be seen when analysing two of the most successful ever tennis stars – left-handed John McEnroe and right-handed Björn Borg (Ditty 2001). McEnroe was famous for his complete inability to keep emotionally cool in a match (making full use of the area of his brain associated with emotional and direct language!). Borg was the complete opposite, renowned for his cool, emotional indifference when under pressure.

The difference between the two brain hemispheres can actually be seen in the face. By splitting a photograph of someone's face in half and then matching the two mirror images with themselves, the resulting portraits (as shown in the three photographs with myself as the subject) illustrate two distinctly different characters. That said, both sides appear to communicate continuously and are able to integrate harmoniously in order to perform very complex tasks.

On a more serious note, the biggest difference between hemisphere function seems to be related to language, and this is an important issue for many people whose lives are affected by stroke. It is the left side of the cerebrum that controls the ability to speak and to communicate using language in nearly all right-handed people, and in some left-handed individuals.

As I mentioned previously, the brain has specific parts devoted to specific functions, and in addition to the hemisphere divide the cerebrum is often further mapped into a number of geographical areas known as lobes (see Figure 8.1) with each lobe having its own function. In addition, there

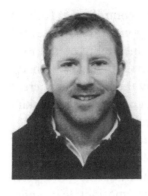 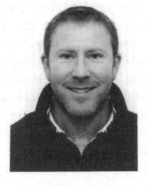 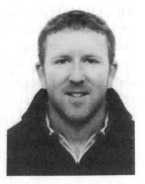

Normal (well, unaltered!)   *Me with two left sides*   *Me with two right sides*

are the other distinct parts of the brain that I named earlier in Figure 7.3. So, the control of appetite and thirst, the registering of fear, the translation of sounds into speech, the processing of vision into colour and images, the control of sleep patterns, and the recognition and distinguishing of faces and objects are all controlled by specific parts of the brain.

Under the cerebrum, or white matter, lie the basal portions of the brain. These are:

- the basal ganglia that interact with the motor portions of the cortex
- the limbic system (which is further divided)
- the cerebellum that controls movement.

The basal ganglia

The basal ganglia are three large masses of cells (ganglia) that lie at the base of the cerebral cortex and surround the thalamus. The basal ganglia, together with the cerebellum and the motor cortex, are responsible for aspects of motor control. Motor commands initiated by the cortex are modified and processed by the basal ganglia. This part of the brain helps the cerebral cortex to execute subconscious and learned movements. It determines how large or small, and how fast or slow, a movement needs to be for optimum performance. The basal ganglia, therefore, is likely to contribute to the control of tremor and ballistic movements.

The blood supply to the basal ganglia is via the middle cerebral artery.

The limbic system

The limbic system evolved within the cerebrum, after 10 million years of evolution, approximately 150 million years ago. In addition to governing activities associated with self-preservation (the famous 'flight or fight' response), the limbic system appears to be responsible for our emotional life. It is said that with the development of the limbic system came a 'social co-operation' within animal species. Damage to the limbic system can cause emotional unrest and dramatic and serious changes in mood.

The limbic system contains several structures, which work collectively, linking body and mind:

- the thalamus
- the hypothalamus
- the amygdala
- the hippocampus.

The thalamus is the inner chamber of the brain and is closely integrated with the cerebral cortex. It is the first stop for all incoming signals to the brain; it is where sensation is first consciously experienced or felt; and it is responsible for the initial processing of all sensory information (with the exception of smell). Blood supply to the thalamus is via the anterior or carotid arterial system.

The hypothalamus is one of the smallest (the size of a pea and about 1/300 of the total brain weight) but busiest parts of the brain. It is mainly concerned with homeostasis through the regulation of the autonomic nervous system (ANS). The hypothalamus controls appetite, sexual arousal, thirst and temperature. It works closely with the pituitary gland (this is situated at the base of the brain and is another pea-sized part), which controls the endocrine system (see p.55). While the endocrine system is generally described in general and introductory textbooks in isolation of the nervous system, in reality the two systems are interdependent. Blood supply to the hypothalamus is from the internal carotid arteries, which lead to the Circle of Willis.

The amygdala controls our defensive behaviour, and processes our emotional memories. It assesses sensory information for threat, and responds by initiating the 'fight or flight' messages to the body. The amygdala alerts the areas of the cerebral cortex connected with fear, anger and sadness. Without it we would be without any emotional response to situations. Blood supply to the amygdala is through the anterior carotid arterial system.

The hippocampus is the brain's memory centre. It has a lot to do with the formation of memories (short-term ones in particular) and is where we store 'unemotional facts'. The hippocampus does not fully develop until early childhood, which explains why we do not really have memories from this time of our lives. As a result of the unique features of its pyramidal cell structure, the hippocampus is one of the first sites of the brain to be irreversibly damaged by an ischaema or a lack of oxygen (anoxia). It is also affected by Alzheimer's disease, which is illustrated by the fact that a sufferer will soon lose short-term memories. Blood supply to the hippocampus is primarily from branches of the posterior cerebral artery.

The cerebellum

The cerebellum developed 70 million years before the cerebrum, and 80 million years before the limbic system. The cerebellum is positioned at the back of the skull below the cerebral hemispheres and above the brainstem and looks a little like two small plums. It is labelled in Figure 7.4; but again, you may find it useful to look ahead at Figure 7.6. The cerebellum oversees and co-ordinates muscle movement and develops what is commonly referred to as 'muscle memory'.

Unlike the cerebral hemispheres, each side of the cerebellum is actually involved with the side of the body that it is situated on. That is, nerve pathways connect the right half of the cerebellum with the left cerebral hemisphere and the right side of the body. Correspondingly, pathways from the left half connect with the right cerebral hemisphere and the left side of the body.

Even though it is very much associated with movement, the cerebellum does not generate movement. Rather, it operates entirely at a subconscious level, working in conjunction with the basal ganglia and the motor portion of the cerebral cortex to make controlled, co-ordinated and balanced motor movements. It communicates with the vestibular system (linked with balance and the ear) and controls the axial muscles of the body, which help to control balance. The cerebellum has been compared to the control centre of a guided missile, which ensures that the missile lands exactly on target.

The cerebellum consists of three sections, which connect to the brainstem in a way similar to a three-pin plug. The first, the vestibulo-cerebellum, is found in all vertebrates and works in close association with the inner ear and is responsible for maintaining the body's orientation in space, balance and posture and also regulates locomotion and other movements, keeping objects in visual focus as the body moves. It is connected to the brainstem via bundles of nerve fibre tracts, or penduncles, entering and exiting the cerebellum. The second section, the spino-cerebellum, automatically interprets information from the spinal cord and is concerned with co-ordinating the planning and timing of movement and correcting deviations in movement. It does the latter by comparing one movement with another and fine-tuning subsequent movements. The ponto-cerebellum is the third and largest section and relates to more skilled or complex movements.

Blood supply to the cerebellum is via the posterior or vertebral arterial system.

The brainstem

The brainstem is the oldest and deepest part of the human brain (it is labelled in Figure 7.6). It developed some 40 million years before the cerebellum, making it around 270 million years old. It has been present in reptiles for 500 million years, and as such is often called the 'reptilian brain'. The brainstem cannot think, feel or offer an emotional response. It simply monitors external sensory information and controls many involuntary functions, such as regulating heart rate. The brainstem consists of the following sections:

- the midbrain
- the pons
- the medulla oblongata

The midbrain is the smallest region of the brainstem. Included in its role are hearing and visual reflexes, such as turning the eyes and tracking objects. The pons informs the cerebellum of what the cerebrum intends during voluntary activity. It is part of a feedback-loop system that the cerebellum employs to co-ordinate and refine muscular activity. In addition, there is a respiratory centre in the pons, which controls expiration of air. The medulla oblongata connects the brain to the very top of the spinal cord. It has a variety of 'centres' and controls many of the involuntary actions of our bodies, such as the regulation of heartbeat, breathing, blood pressure, swallowing, vomiting, sneezing, coughing and digestion.

Basic vessel anatomy for the lay person

Stroke occurs, as we have already established, as the result of an abnormal supply of blood to, or within, the brain. The exact consequences of the ischaemia or haemorrhage will depend upon which areas are affected.

Clearly, in order to better understand this and how the normal blood supply to the brain can be interrupted, we really need to understand how the blood supplies the brain.

Blood travels continuously around the body through the circulatory system, which is powered by a pump – the heart. The oxygen-rich (oxygenated) blood travels in arteries away from the heart. The oxygen-depleted (de-oxygenated) blood returns to the heart by way of the veins. Like all organs, the brain is dependent on oxygenated blood travelling from the heart. The brain itself is supplied with blood by two kinds of arteries (sometimes referred to as arterial territories), and in a healthy person some 740 millilitres of blood circulate around the brain every minute.

Blood is supplied to the brain by first travelling through the aorta (the main artery from the heart) and up through the aortic arch into one of four arteries (these are actually two pairs). These are known as the carotid arteries and vertebral arteries, which all pass up the neck and lead to the brain. They are, to some extent, all evident in Figures 7.4, 7.6 and 8.1. However, a slightly more detailed representation of blood flow to, and within, the brain can be seen in my flowchart (Figure 7.5).

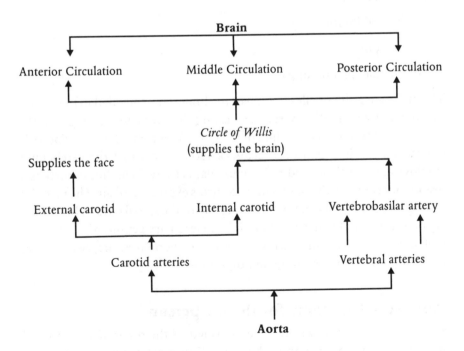

Figure 7.5: A simplified circulatory pathway of blood to the brain

As Figure 7.5 illustrates, the carotid arteries branch into the internal and external carotid arteries, and the vertebral arteries join together to form the vertebrobasilar artery. While the external carotid arteries supply the face with blood, the internal carotid artery and vertebrobasilar artery meet and feed what is known as the interior brain artery, which is called the Circle of Willis.

When at the brain, the blood supply is routed through branching arteries that enter the brain in order to supply specific areas. This system of arteries is called the cerebral artery system. The cerebral artery system can be further divided into anterior, posterior and middle circulations based on the area of the brain that part of the system supplies. Simply speaking, there are six major cerebral arteries with one on each side of the brain, leading either to the front, rear or middle part of the brain. In addition, the brain has a drainage system of de-oxygenated blood through a system of veins. However, I won't go into detail about these here.

The middle and anterior circulation of blood

The carotid arteries

The carotid arteries are the two main vessels in the neck that run up the side of the neck and carry blood to the head and brain. As I have said above, the external carotid arteries supply the face with blood, and any blockage or clotting problems in here will obviously not lead to a stroke. It is, therefore, the internal carotid arteries that are really of interest in matters relating to strokes. The internal carotid arteries supply the anterior and middle parts of the cerebral hemispheres, the basal ganglia, limbic system and eye. Some mention should be made to the ophthalmic artery (this feeds the eye) when discussing strokes, as damage to the ophthalmic artery can result in blind spots, a loss of vision in one eye, a loss of half of vision in both eyes, or a number of variations of these.

It is largely as the result of the meandering route of the internal carotid arteries that cholesterol can build up and blockages may occur. The internal carotid arteries are, therefore, frequently the site of a blockage caused by atherosclerotic disease. Among the branches off the internal carotid arteries are two main branches, which are known as the middle and anterior cerebral arteries. These arteries supply the frontal, temporal and parietal lobes with blood.

The middle cerebral arteries

The middle cerebral arteries are actually the most common arteries involved in stroke. Because they supply so much of the brain with blood, an interruption in blood flow can cause numerous disorders. Some branches of the middle cerebral arteries (the striata) are even known as the 'arteries of stroke'. Due to the very thin walls, but relatively high pressure within the walls, these particular arteries are more susceptible to haemorrhaging than blockage. That said, blockages within the system of the middle arteries are the most common cause of stroke.

A blockage in the middle cerebral arteries may cause a stroke resulting in contralateral (opposite) paralysis that affects the arm, the lower part of the face, speech and swallowing. As the middle cerebral artery supplies the entire lateral hemispheres with blood, depending on the hemisphere affected, a blockage causing a stroke may also result in language and cognition deficits, and problems with swallowing, smell and hearing.

The anterior cerebral artery

The anterior cerebral artery is the second most common artery involved in stroke. A blockage of the anterior cerebral arteries causing stroke may result in sensory and motor impairment of the legs and lower body (including the bowel and bladder), and dyspraxia (see Glossary). In addition, as they also supply blood to the frontal lobes, a stroke involving the anterior cerebral arteries may result in problems with reasoning and understanding, and some associated language impairment.

The posterior circulation of blood

The vertebral arteries

The vertebral arteries are smaller than the carotid arteries and run up alongside the spinal column. The left and right vertebral arteries have a number of branches off them, as do the internal carotid arteries, which lead to the cerebellum. The left and right vertebral arteries then join together to form the vertebrobasilar artery. This has further branches off it. Unlike the internal carotid arteries, the vertebral and vertebrobasilar arteries are quite straight and not as prone to the build-up of cholesterol and blockages in the way that the internal carotid arteries are. However, they can haemorrhage or suffer a dissection. I have already mentioned the causes of dissection in Part I, but discuss this in more detail later.

The vertebrobasilar arteries supply blood to the posterior parts of the cerebral hemispheres, including the occipital lobes, the posterior portions

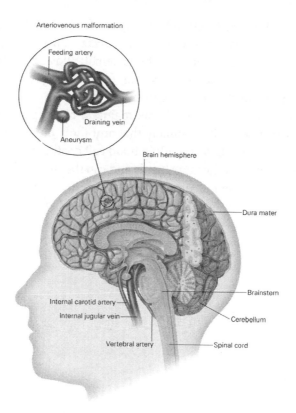

Figure 7.6: Side view of the brain showing normal blood vessels, and an enlarged section showing an arteriovenous malformation and an aneurysm. Illustration by Philip Wilson FMAA RMIP. Reproduced with permission from the Brain and Spine Foundation.

of the temporal lobes, the limbic system, the cerebellum, brainstem and spinal cord. This vertebrobasilar system deals largely with the vital functions. However, a stroke involving the vertebral arteries and vertebrobasilar system can also result in visual defects (perception and field), memory loss and language disorders. Specifically, if the branch supplying the midbrain is affected, the result may include motor abnormalities. If the branch supplying the thalamus is affected, then pain may also be a significant issue.

The Circle of Willis

I have said previously that all the arteries supplying blood to the brain arise from the aortic arch. The two internal carotid arteries and the vertebrobasilar arteries meet at the base of the brain and form what is called the Circle of Willis. The Circle of Willis is, in effect, a circular, interior brain artery that has branches that travel to the surface of the cerebral cortex, interior of the brain, cerebellum and brainstem. It allows blood to pass from the carotid and vertebral arteries and can, to some extent, provide a safety mechanism if one of the arteries gets blocked.

Providing the Circle of Willis can maintain blood pressure at 50 per cent of its normal level, it is unlikely that any short interruption in blood flow within these vessels will result in brain cell death. However, with age, these blood vessels become more brittle and can themselves be a significant cause of stroke in some individuals.

Chapter 8

The Stroke: Signs, Symptoms and Causes

A physiological warning of stroke – transient ischaemic attack

The most common warning sign of stroke is the *transient ischaemic attack* (TIA). A TIA is often referred to as a 'mini-stroke', and is a short period of disturbance of body function, lasting for less than 24 hours, resulting from a temporary reduction in blood supply to part of the brain. Depending on the area of the brain affected by a TIA, the sufferer can have a temporary loss of limb sensation or strength, a loss of vision, or even a loss of consciousness. A TIA commonly lasts between two and 15 minutes, and having been rapid in its onset leaves no persistent neurological deficit. However, TIAs must always be taken seriously no matter how quickly they pass, as they are a clear warning that a life-threatening stroke may occur soon.

TIAs should always be investigated, the cause should be found and, if possible, treated. Without treatment, about one in four people who have had a TIA will have a stroke within the next few years. It is therefore quite clear that each and every TIA should be taken seriously, by both the individual concerned and those members of the medical profession he or she presents to. It is not too late to seek medical attention or advice even when the symptoms have gone away.

The important emphasis in terms of identifying the cause of a stroke is that, if at all possible, it should be done *before* the stroke happens, in a proactive, preventative way, and not afterwards in a reactive, rehabilitative way. However, until the general population take some responsibility for themselves, scientists are still trying to develop and improve risk-score methods to predict, and aim to prevent, a stroke. The Oxford Stroke Prevention Research Unit has identified four factors that could predict the future risk of a stroke if an individual suffers and reports a TIA. These are:

1.   the **A**ge of the individual

2.   the **B**lood pressure of the individual

3.   the **C**linical features (i.e. the symptoms) the individual presents

4.   the **D**uration of the TIA.

Simply speaking, by translating these facts to create an ABCD score, the high-risk individuals, who may need emergency treatment, can be identified. The majority of TIAs are the result of arterial or cardiac thromboses, but they may equally be associated with high blood pressure, smoking, obesity, high cholesterol levels, or a combination of all of these.

The onset of stroke

The primary identifying feature of stroke is its acute and sudden onset. In other words, the symptoms of stroke happen immediately. In rare cases, these symptoms of a stroke can be difficult to attribute to a stroke with any certainty, even for doctors. However, this is not usually the case, and a failure to identify the symptoms of a stroke in another is really the result of poor education or ignorance caused by complacency. In a 1996 Gallup survey conducted for the National Stroke Association, 17 per cent of adults over age 50 were unable to name a single stroke symptom. Unfortunately such a lack of awareness can spell disaster. The stroke victim may suffer significant brain damage when people nearby fail to recognise the symptoms of a stroke.

As I have discussed, each part of the brain has more than one specific function and each part of the brain can be subject to a stroke. As a result, the general and most common symptoms of stroke include:

- numbness or weakness in the face, arms or legs (especially on one side of the body)
- confusion, difficulty speaking or understanding speech
- vision disturbances in one or both eyes
- dizziness
- some trouble walking
- a loss of balance or co-ordination
- a severe headache with no known cause.

While the symptoms may be inconsistent, depending on the area of the brain affected by the interruption in normal blood flow, there can be no doubt of the following – the longer blood flow is cut off to the brain, the greater the potential for permanent damage to the brain. Within a few minutes of the onset of a stroke, the area of the brain affected is damaged, some of it beyond repair.

Any observer can recognise a possible stroke by asking the following three simple questions of the person suffering:

1.   Can you raise your arms and keep them up?

2.   Can you smile?

3.   Can you repeat a simple sentence?

If the answer to one or more of these questions is 'no', then immediate medical attention should be sought. If the individual in distress has in fact had a stroke, the full and lasting effects, as I have said, will be dependent upon the area of the brain affected and the speed with which medical attention is given.

Why stroke occurs

I have mentioned previously that a stroke occurs when a blood clot blocks a blood vessel or artery, or when a blood vessel breaks, interrupting blood flow to an area of the brain. It most often occurs when the carotid arteries become blocked and the brain does not get enough oxygen. The physical damage depends upon which blood vessel is damaged and whether the damage was due to blockage or haemorrhage.

Stroke caused by a blockage or clot – ischaemia

In everyday life, blood clotting is most beneficial. When an individual bleeds from a wound, blood clots work to slow and eventually stop the bleeding. In the case of a stroke, however, blood clots are dangerous because they can block arteries and cut off blood flow. Ischaemic strokes can happen as the result of unhealthy blood vessels, which are clogged with a build-up of fatty deposits and cholesterol. This condition is known as 'atherosclerosis'. The body regards atherosclerosis as multiple, tiny and repeated injuries to the blood vessel wall. It then reacts to these injuries just as if it was bleeding from a wound, and it responds by forming clots. Atherosclerosis is often associated with stroke and the supply of blood to the brain, and is the progressive narrowing and hardening of arteries over time. It is known to occur with ageing, but other factors include high cholesterol, high blood pressure, smoking, diabetes and a family history of athero-sclerotic disease. Other causes of ischaemic stroke include use of street drugs, traumatic injury to the blood vessels of the neck, or disorders of blood clotting.

Approximately 80 per cent of all strokes are ischaemic. Due to the con-tributory factors of ischaemic stroke mentioned above, many people who suffer them are older (60 or more years old), and the risk of ischaemic stroke increases with age.

As I clarified earlier, an ischaemic stroke can occur in two ways, and will then often be classified as an 'embolic' or a 'thrombotic' stroke. This is illus-trated very clearly in Figure 8.1.

Embolic stroke

With an embolic stroke, a blood clot forms somewhere in the body and then moves. This kind of blockage causing a stroke is called a 'cerebral embolism'. While it may form in the arteries of the chest and neck, a part may break off before travelling through the bloodstream to the brain. Alternatively, it may possibly form in the heart, but again a part may break off and travel to the brain.

Once in the brain, the clot eventually travels through the system until it reaches a blood vessel small enough to block its passage. When it can travel no further, the clot lodges there blocking the blood vessel and causing a stroke.

Thrombotic stroke

In the case of a thrombotic stroke, blood flow is impaired because of a blockage that has built up in one or more of the arteries supplying blood to the brain, most often in the large arteries, such as the carotid artery or middle cerebral artery. A significant number of strokes are caused by block-ages and narrowing of the carotid arteries and carotid artery disease increases the risk for stroke in three ways:

- through fatty deposits (cholesterol or plaque) building up and severely narrowing the carotid arteries

- by a blood clot becoming stuck in a carotid artery, which has already been narrowed by plaque

- by plaque breaking off from the carotid arteries and in so doing blocking one of the smaller arteries in the brain (cerebral artery).

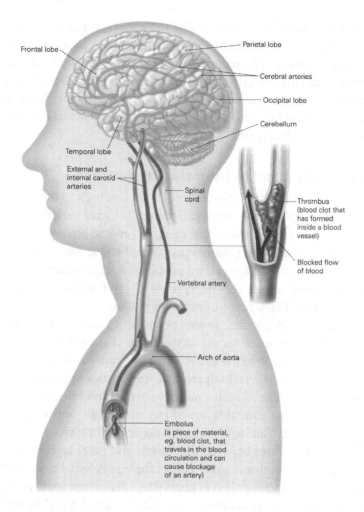

Figure 8.1: The main blood supply to the brain; the enlarged section shows blockage of the artery, which can cause a stroke. Illustration by Philip Wilson FMAA RMIP. Reproduced with permission from the Brain and Spine Foundation.

Generally speaking, if a carotid artery is blocked then a cerebral stroke will result. If a vertebral artery is blocked, then a cerebellar or brainstem stroke will result. The process leading to this blockage is what is known as thrombosis, and there are two types of thrombosis which can cause a stroke – large vessel thrombosis and small vessel disease.

Large vessel thrombosis is the most common, and probably the most understood type of thrombotic stroke. Most large vessel thrombosis is caused by a combination of long-term atherosclerosis, followed by a rapid blood clot formation. It is common that thrombotic stroke patients are also likely to have coronary artery disease, and actually a heart attack is a frequent cause of death in patients who have suffered this type of stroke.

Small vessel disease (also called lacunar infarction) occurs when the blood flow is blocked to a very small, but often a deep, penetrating, arterial vessel. Very little is known about the causes of small vessel disease, but it seems to be very closely linked to hypertension.

Ischaemic stroke caused by cervical artery dissection

In order to fully understand this section, I refer you back to the information on the blood supply to the brain in Chapter 7. I have included this additional section for two reasons. First, because cervical artery dissection is a common cause of stroke in younger people and stroke must not be considered to be purely an (old) age-related problem (despite what has been mentioned previously about the likely causes); and second, because this explains the most likely cause of my own stroke.

It seems that a dissection, or tear, occurs in an area of an artery where there is weakness for some reason. In the study of strokes, the artery is carrying blood and oxygen to the brain, and dissection can therefore occur in the cervical (carotid or vertebral) arteries. Any weakness in the artery wall (or lining), even combined with a normal arterial blood pressure, can result in a separation of the natural layers of the artery wall, and some blood is then pushed from its usual route through the artery. In such cases, the blood may deviate into an area between the middle and inner layer of the artery, or even cause a new pathway along part of the vessel. Some blood then clots in the arterial wall causing what is known as a dissecting aneurysm. It may act as a tourniquet, or subsequently be dislodged and travel to the brain, resulting in a stroke.

Even though this cause of stroke is uncommon, it is an increasingly recognised condition. Nevertheless, it is important to mention that dissections may not always lead to stroke. Who is susceptible to dissection, and what the outcome on the body may be, is unpredictable.

A cervical arterial dissection can be categorised as the result of:

- an event resulting in direct trauma to the neck
- a spontaneous event
- a precipitating event.

Both vertebral artery dissection (VAD) and carotid artery dissection (CAD) are increasingly recognised causes of strokes in young patients. Usually, due to the general absence of arteriosclerosis (see Glossary) in the young, VAD and CAD are the underlying cause in as many as 20 per cent of the ischaemic strokes suffered by those aged 30–45 years.

The average age for VAD is just 40 years old, while the average age of a patient with CAD is just 47 years old. While CAD is three to five times more common than VAD, the latter has been associated with a 10 per cent mortality rate in the acute phase.

Because I had some of the pre-stroke (even though they were relatively mild) symptoms associated with VAD, and because I experienced an acute onset (this was anything but mild!) with a sudden loss of functions and suffered a cerebellar stroke, my stroke consultant believes that I survived a VAD, even in the absence of a definitive vascular MRI scan. What caused the VAD remains unknown.

To elaborate, such dissections can be caused by participation in sport and similar activities, chiropractic manipulation, painting ceilings, coughing, sneezing, whiplash or, occasionally, simply by turning the head. The vertebral artery follows a slightly twisting path into the skull and is, therefore, especially vulnerable to damage as a result of torsion or twisting. As I mentioned in Part I, such cervical artery dissection is even known by some as 'beauty parlour syndrome'. This is due to the fact that, in some cases, it is known to have been the result of an individual leaning their head backwards over a sink in order to have their hair washed.

With specific regard to chiropractic manipulation, which is undoubtedly an effective therapy for head and neck pain, it may be advisable to avoid it if the pain is the result of a specific injury-causing event, especially that involving the rotation of the head. There are definite recorded cases of neck manipulation resulting in cervical artery dissection leading to stroke. In fact, my own stroke consultant referred to such a case in one of our consultations.

Stroke caused by bleeding – haemorrhage

In the case of a haemorrhagic stroke, which accounts for the remaining 20 per cent of strokes after ischaemic strokes, it is, as I have already said, the breakage of a blood vessel in the brain that leads to bleeding. The bleeding then irritates the brain tissue and causes swelling (known as cerebral oedema). The surrounding tissues of the brain resist the bleeding, which can be contained by forming a mass (haematoma). Both swelling and haematoma will compress and displace normal brain tissue causing damage.

Haemorrhages can be caused by a number of disorders, which affect the blood vessels, including long-standing hypertension (high blood pressure), high cholesterol and cerebral aneurysms (see Glossary). A cerebral aneurysm, usually present at birth, can develop over a number of years and may not cause a detectable problem until it breaks. As I clarified earlier, there are two categories of stroke caused by haemorrhage – subarachnoid and intracerebral.

In a subarachnoid haemorrhage (SAH), an aneurysm bursts in a large artery on or near the thin, delicate membrane surrounding the brain. Blood then spills into the area around the brain causing a stroke. This tends to be managed very differently from other strokes. Bleeding may recur within weeks and there is a far greater chance that surgery will be needed to repair the artery. In the case of an intracerebral haemorrhage, bleeding occurs from vessels within the brain itself. As I stated earlier, hypertension is the primary cause of this type of haemorrhage.

Chapter 9

After a Stroke

The effects of stroke

Trying to summarise all the possible effects of a stroke under one heading is close to an impossible task. There are simply too many individual factors, which vary from individual to individual, to take into account. In my opinion, the important issues regarding the effects of a stroke become really evident with the answers to these questions:

- Why…has a stroke occurred?

- How…could an individual be affected?

- Who…is available to support recovery?

- What…can be implemented to aid with recovery, or improve the quality of life for all those affected?

The Why? has been discussed above. The How? is discussed below. The Who? and What? are both considered in later chapters.

The specific abilities that will be lost or affected by stroke depend on:

- the extent of the brain damage

- where in the brain the stroke occurred.

In order to begin to appreciate how an individual can be affected having survived a stroke, I think that our knowledge of how the brain works should be applied. Therefore, I have decided to include an overview of the most common effects first by hemisphere, and then by individual sections of the brain.

Hemisphere strokes

Possible effects of a right-sided stroke:

- Movement and mobility: left hemiplegia (see Glossary), and some spatial and perceptual problems.

- Vision: inability to see the left visual field of each eye.

- One-sided neglect: ignoring objects or individuals to the left.

- Behaviour: judgement difficulties. This is often displayed through impulsive behaviour, where the individual may ignore any disability and try to complete the same tasks as before the stroke. It can also extend to 'inappropriate' behaviour.

- Memory: short-term memory loss.

- Emotional health: depression.

In addition, persistent talking may be the result of right lobe damage.

Possible effects of a left-sided stroke:

- Movement and mobility: right hemiplegia (see Glossary).

- Vision: inability to see the right visual field of each eye.

- Language: if the part known as Wernicke's area is affected this may result in problems with understanding language; and if the part known as Broca's area (situated close by) is affected, this may result in problems with speech.

- Behaviour: judgement difficulties, but in contrast to a right-sided stroke, the individual may require frequent instruction and feedback, thereby becoming slower and more cautious.

- Memory: increased problems with learning new tasks. In addition, paying attention, conceptualising and generalising may be difficult.

- Emotional health: depression.

Effects on different lobes

In order to be a little more specific, once again it is worth considering dividing the hemispheres into lobes. Lehr's (1998) presentation paper, which maps brain function, explains this well and I have adapted it for the purposes of this book.

Table 9.1 summarises the functions and possible problems related to the given lobe and, again, you may find it useful to check the location of the lobe with Figure 8.1.

Table 9.1 Functions of and possible problems related to different lobes

Area of cerebral cortex and location	Its functions	Possible problems after stroke
Frontal lobe (located under forehead)	Front portion	Difficulty in persevering with a single thought
	Conscious thought	Inability to plan a sequence of complex movements needed to complete multi-stepped tasks, e.g. making a mug of tea
	Initiating activity in response to the environment	Difficulty in problem solving
	Control of emotional responses	Difficulty in interacting with others
	Memory habits	Changes in social behaviour
	Control of expressive language	Changes in personality
	Giving meaning to words (involving word associations)	Loss of flexibility in thinking
		Inability to focus on task
	Rear portion	Mood changes
	Involved in the production of movement	Inability to express language (Broca's aphasia)
		Paralysis of specific body parts
Parietal lobe (located at top of the head, near back)	Aspects of the sensation of touch (pressure, size, texture, weight, shape)	Lack of awareness of certain body parts and/or surrounding space (apraxia) that can lead to difficulties in self-care
	Right parietal lobe	Inability to recognise objects (agnosia)
	Interpretation of visual/spatial information	Inability to name an object (anomia)
	Left parietal lobe	Inability to locate the words for writing (agraphia)
	Spoken and written language	Problems with reading (alexia)
		Difficulty with doing mathematics (dyscalculia)
		Difficulty with drawing objects
		Difficulty in distinguishing left from right
		Inability to focus visual attention
		Difficulties with eye and hand co-ordination

Table 9.1 continued

Occipital lobe (located at the back of the head)	The area for visual reception and the processing of visual information including shapes and colours	Defects in vision (visual field cuts), including inaccurately seeing objects Difficulty with locating objects in the environment Difficulty with identifying colours (colour agnosia) Word blindness – inability to recognise words Difficulty in recognising drawn objects Inability to recognise the movement of an object (movement agnosia) Difficulties with reading and writing Hallucinations

Temporal lobe (located above ears, on side of head)	Include distinguishing different sounds and different smells
	Right temporal lobe
	    Visual memory
	Left temporal lobe
	    Verbal memory
		Difficulty in recognising faces (prosopagnosia)
		Difficulty in understanding spoken words (Wernicke's aphasia)
		Disturbance with selective attention to what is seen and heard
		Difficulty with identifying and describing objects
		Inability to categorise objects
		Short-term memory loss
		Long-term memory problems
		Changed (decreased or increased) interest in sexual behaviour
		Increased aggressive behaviour
		NB. Right lobe damage, specifically, can cause persistent talking

Left-sided stroke and speech

As I have already said, speech problems are commonly associated with a stroke, and so I think it is worth exploring this aspect of the effects of a stroke a little further. While it is not inevitable that speech problems will be the result of damage to the left hemisphere, it is the left hemisphere that is most closely concerned with language. Damage to the anterior part of the cerebrum can cause 'non-fluent disorders' (also known as Broca's aphasia) while damage to the posterior part can cause the fluent type (also known as Wernicke's aphasia).

Sufferers of non-fluent aphasia find it difficult to recall words (particularly more uncommon words) and name objects. They may insert swear words or some taboo words while trying to think of the words that they cannot remember. In addition, they will very likely find it difficult to talk fluently and will often be frustrated as they will actually be acutely aware of the hesitation in speech. Therefore, some physicians and therapists believe that the difficulty here is more the result of the loss of the ability to find the right words at the right moment than the actual loss of the ability to talk.

By contrast, the fluent aphasiac's intonation will be quite normal but the words and context will probably be meaningless. Unlike the non-fluent aphasiac, the fluent aphasiac will be unlikely to realise the communication difficulties. Similarly, while it may be possible that reading, writing and comprehension difficulties may be present in both types of patient, all are generally more severe in fluent aphasiacs.

Effects on other brain areas following a stroke

Basal ganglia disorders

The most noticeable disorders to this area following a stroke are:

- motor control problems rather than motor weakness

- too much movement, or 'hyperkinesia' (as displayed by sufferers of chorea: involuntary, dance-like movement of the extremities and head)

- too little movement, or 'hypokinesia' (as displayed by sufferers of Parkinson's disease).

Disorders of the thalamus

A person may experience thalamic pain, sometimes referred to as 'central pain syndrome', due to damage to the spinal tracts that carry pain and temperature sensation to the thalamus. Thalamic pain usually starts several weeks after the stroke and presents as an intense burning pain on the side of the body affected by the stroke.

Disorders of the cerebellum

Although, as I have said previously, strokes are less common in the cerebellum, the effects can be severe. A stroke affecting the cerebellum will cause disruption in balance, and in the timing and force of movement. The following symptoms are commonly seen in cases of cerebellar stroke:

- ataxia – lack of motor co-ordination due to irregularities in timing, rate and force of muscular contraction

- unsteady gait – displayed by grossly unco-ordinated or 'drunken' gait

- loss of balance and a tendency to fall

- dizziness – specifically a sensation of spinning and nausea

- intention tremor – tremor, which worsens with movement

- dysdiadochokinesia – the inability to perform rapid, alternating movements

- dysmetria – the overshoot or undershoot of a movement evident in inability to reach out and grab objects

- pendular swinging of a joint – a large swinging movement after joint displacement (for example, after a patellar tendon tap)

- nystagmus – conjugate drift of the gaze followed by rapid return to the centre

- disruption to the normal flow and rhythm of speech (scanning speech)

- decrease in muscle tone and stretch reflex.

Disorders of the brainstem – medulla, the pons and midbrain

As the brainstem is the area of the brain that controls all of our involuntary 'life-support' functions (such as breathing rate, blood pressure and heartbeat), it is obvious that strokes that occur in the brainstem are especially devastating. In addition, the brainstem also controls abilities such as eye movements, hearing, speech and swallowing. Since impulses generated in the brain's hemispheres must travel through the brainstem on their way to the arms and legs, patients with a brainstem stroke may also develop paralysis in one or both sides of the body. Unfortunately, death is common in the case of brainstem strokes.

Cervical artery dissection and stroke

A sudden, severe neck pain is the identifying feature of a cervical arterial dissection. This can often prove useful in identifying when the dissection took place as it may occur some hours, days or possibly weeks before the onset of stroke. I think that it is worth repeating in this context that some doctors do not believe that arterial dissection will automatically lead to stroke and certainly not death. What the medical profession do agree on is that any initial pain that is then followed by a period of continued neck pain is a reliable symptom of dissection.

A stroke caused by a cervical arterial dissection follows the typical path and destination of the artery. Therefore:

- CAD (carotid artery dissection) can cause weakness on one side of the body (hemiparesis), hemisensory loss and other cerebral hemispheric features such as aphasia

- VAD (vertebrobasilar artery dissection) may result in ataxia and a severe or complete loss of motor function in all four limbs (quadriparesis).

Prognosis following stroke

A lack of understanding, or an inaccurate diagnosis of the underlying cause of a physical problem, can lead to inadequate and sometimes non-existent treatment options in the case of a stroke. That said, this certainly did not happen in my case, even though I presented one of the more rare cases. While recovery after stroke can be slow, difficult and sometimes only partial, I repeat that it is very clear that there is a need for immediate medical attention if a stroke is suspected. Even a small stroke (in terms of how it is displayed on a brain scan) can result in a major loss of function if it happens in one of the more 'vital' parts of the brain. Often patients with relatively mild symptoms actually delay calling for the doctor, or going to the hospital, and so miss the opportunity to have early treatment, which may have proved to be very effective!

Following a stroke, there is usually an area around the most severely damaged part of the brain that is only partly affected. When brain cells in the infarct die, they release chemicals that set off a chain reaction called the 'ischaemic cascade'. This chain reaction endangers brain cells in a larger, surrounding area of brain tissue for which the blood supply is compromised but not completely cut off (see Figure 7.4). Without prompt medical treatment this larger area of brain cells will also die.

Due to the rapid pace of the ischaemic cascade, the time for interventional treatment is limited to about six hours. Any longer than this and the re-establishment of blood flow and the administration of chemical treatment may not only fail to help, but may also cause further damage. Unfortunately, around 42 per cent of stroke patients wait as much as 24 hours before presenting themselves for medical treatment, which is at least 18 hours too late! In terms of a thrombotic stroke, such a delay results in a missed opportunity to effectively treat the damage caused.

When a stroke has been confirmed, the aim of initial treatment and care is to *minimise* the area of permanent damage and *protect* the penumbra, so that all subsequent treatment and care may include encouraging the healthy part of the brain to take over from the damaged cells. As I have said previously, damaged nerve tissue is not thought to regenerate, but in terms of damage to the brain (including damage as the result of stroke) there seems to be a flexible system that can allow a range of recovery in function. The medical profession does not fully understand how this happens, but it may be due in part to the interconnectedness of the nerve cells within the brain and central nervous system. It seems that a damaged brain is sometimes able to reorganise itself and may recover some function, as long as there is some continued sensory input. This development of nerve pathways is called 'neuroplasticity'. For example, if the stroke was caused by a blocked artery, and we know from the study of the blood supply to the brain that there is some overlap between the areas of the brain supplied by the arteries, then some parts of the area affected may still survive (albeit with less blood).

There are a variety of issues, including age, gender differences, and function, which affect neuroplasticity. For example, it seems that the younger brain recovers more readily than the older brain; and women may be more successful than men in combating language problems associated with left-sided stroke. One reason for this could be that a greater proportion of women seem to have language abilities in both hemispheres.

However, the rate of potential and actual progress following a stroke is also uncertain. A few days after the stroke most people have a fast period of recovery, which then begins to slow down. However, other stroke survivors make little progress for many weeks and then suddenly display signs of improvement. In terms of the limbs, movement in the leg may start recovery before the arm. Similarly, swallowing difficulties may significantly improve within a month while speech difficulties may not begin to improve for some time, and yet then continue to improve after many other functions have stopped improving. Regarding speech, an important factor appears to be the degree to which a person made use of language before the stroke. What is important for all stroke survivors, however, is that there is evidence that recovery in function can still occur two years after the stroke.

I would obviously urge anyone to seek medical advice if their lifestyle leaves them susceptible to having a stroke. I found it hard enough to cope with having had a stroke and I did not have any clearly identifiable health risk factors. Had I been at obvious risk and done nothing, I think that I would have found coming to terms with the experience and the long road to recovery almost unbearable.

Nevertheless, I recognise that some delay in seeking medical advice is certainly understandable. Some people may dismiss their symptoms as too minor to warrant taking up a doctor's time. On reflection, I fell into this category, despite the strange onset of a headache one night. It seems that men, in particular, subconsciously believe that if they ignore a health problem it will just go away! Other people may not go to the doctor for a very different reason. They might just be too scared of what they may find out about themselves if they visit a doctor. Unfortunately, in the case of the latter, it is possible that this itself will lead to further anxiety, which may cause them to increase their susceptibility to the factors that are the very ones of concern – for example, smoking, drinking or overeating.

Clearly, easy access to lifestyle-changing health information that reaches far beyond stroke, perhaps information like that contained in Chapter 10 'A Toolkit for Recovery and Prevention', is vital. However, in terms of stroke specifically, society will benefit from a greater number of people developing a greater awareness of the risk factors, symptoms and need for action relating to stroke. The current outlook for developed societies is not very good because, as a whole, we are failing to recognise the rapid downturn in the general health of the population and are failing to address the consequences of rapidly moving towards an ageing population.

Part III

Surviving Stroke: Ensuring Recovery and Dealing with the Financial Impact

~ Chapter 10 ~

A Toolkit for Recovery and Prevention

My method of recovery: players to the game

My experience of the stroke, and my subsequent research into the 'world of strokes', illustrates one thing very clearly. In recent years, scientific and medical sophistication in assessing and offering immediate treatment to stroke sufferers has grown (and is continuing to improve) but society's ability to prevent a stroke has not kept pace. As recently as the mid-1990s, an American survey illustrated that 38 per cent of Americans aged over 50 did not even know where in the body a stroke occurs, much less what action they could take to prevent one. It is hardly surprising then that inaction in terms of a stroke is commonplace. As I stated clearly in Part II the outcome and recovery of stroke can never be predicted, so prevention is clearly the best option.

My approach to my recovery from stroke, and consequently my attempts to avoid another one (secondary prevention), has been very proactive and remains very much life-centred. Importantly, it is also sustainable and it affords me the opportunity for constant fine-tuning. I call it the 'players to the game' approach.

What is the 'players to the game' approach?

'Players to the game' is a simple, contemporary concept that I have applied to planning, to participating in and to evaluating my recovery from the stroke. It is also one that I am applying in order to take all positive action needed to minimise the risk of ever having another one, although I now know as well as anyone that nothing in life is certain! Before having my stroke, I had long used this concept and approach, with great success, to improving my martial art skill and knowledge and the skill and knowledge of others.

'Players to the game' is a phrase coined by Rick Moneymaker of Virginia, and has been an inspiration to me as he is undoubtedly one of the best martial art instructors in the world. He co-founded the multi-discipline martial art organisation Dragon Society International (DSI), with his partner Tom Muncy, also of Virginia. Use of the 'players to the game' approach helped them to vastly improve the effectiveness of their martial art training methods.

Stated very simply, this concept is split into two parts:

- The *game* – which encompasses all desired outcomes (these can be short-, medium- and/or long-term)

- The *players* – which encompass all aspects that contribute to achieving the outcomes (to use a sporting analogy: the more quality players on your side, the greater your chances of success).

I sincerely hope that this concept will be of value to you, but must stress that for you to use it effectively, the desired outcomes (the game) must first be clearly identified. Then, you must accept that there is no magic route to achieving this desired outcome. With this clearly understood, the factors that can contribute to achieving the desired outcomes can then be considered carefully.

First, you need to decide what your players are. Second, each player should then be subject to scrutiny and questioning in an attempt to fully understand its role. For example, the recovery or prevention of a stroke is not simply a matter of doing everything possible, but rather of prioritising and concentrating on the players that enable you to be most successful. Finally, each player should be identified in order of priority for them to be most effective (the more players and the greater the understanding of the role of each player, the greater the chances of success). This will result in real achievement by way of a multi-disciplinary, productive and energy-efficient programme, and will avoid you wasting your time in unproductive endeavours.

How can the value of each player be assessed?

In order to co-ordinate all the players that were part of my daily routine and in order to evaluate whether they were contributing to my progress I used the fairly well-known SMART targets. Quite simply, I asked a series of questions of each player:

- Were the methods I was employing **S**pecific and my objectives unambiguous?

- Would my objectives by **M**easurable and determined when met?

- Were my objectives **A**chievable?

- Would the success bring sufficient **R**eward to warrant the effort?

- What was my **T**ime frame in order to achieve my objectives?

I found it useful to clearly structure the various aspects of the planning, performing and evaluation of my rehabilitation and stroke prevention programme. To help with this I designed the 'Achievement Log', which shows you two examples of goals, the players used, and whether the goals were achieved:

SMART goal	'Players'	Completion/ Review Date	Achieved
1. walking for 20 mins unaided	Appendicular skeleton, Axial skeleton, Breathing, Components of fitness, Core strength, FITT guidelines, Goal setting and recognising achievement, Kinesiology, Massage therapy, Positive thinking, Posture, Principles of training	1.3.2004	✓
2. take steps to lower cholesterol	Aspirin, Macronutrients, Micronutrients, Nutrition	1.4.2004	✓

This simple log can be easily adapted to suit anyone's programme, and it allows for the SMART goals and players used to be clearly identified. Of course, if a stroke survivor is unable to plan and record such information independently, it may prove a useful aid for a partner, family, friend or carer.

I realise that this is a very disciplined approach, and such an integrated method can get complicated, but my recovery is an issue to which I wanted to commit myself fully, and my future health is something that is of obvious importance to me and those who love and care about me. Furthermore, attempting to recover from a stroke, or engaging in a preventive programme, cannot really be a passive process, and there is evidence that active care following a stroke leads to fewer stroke-related deaths, and less disability for those who survive.

How to select players

The interplay between the complex physiological and emotional experiences which I recounted in Part I illustrates how any rehabilitative programme needs to be both creative and individualised. In addition, the complex nature of stroke as it affects each stroke survivor prevents the application of any single programme for post-stroke rehabilitation. The 'players to the game' approach takes this into account, which is why I believe that it is so appropriate and helpful.

What I really find of most value, especially in the context of looking at stroke and lifestyle, is that the approach can be tailored for each individual, and to his or her own very personal goals. In my case, this allowed for the incorporation of the practice and philosophy of 'integrated medicine and health', which utilises both conventional and more traditional and complementary approaches to the maintenance of good health. This is something that I've always felt to be important – after all, good health is a complete state of physical, social and mental wellbeing and is not merely the absence of disease or infirmity. The integrated approach offers a great way to encourage positive action, using preventive measures to promote the chances of living free from disease. When illness does exist, it seeks to use the best and most appropriate conventional and traditional medical techniques. For some chronic conditions, traditional medicine is recognised as being at least as effective as, and certainly cheaper than, conventional treatment.

'Complementary' approaches

Even before my stroke, I was open to both conventional and some complementary therapies. Now I am even more convinced that they should both be part of healthcare practice and lifestyle advice. The conflict that exists between them is probably an unhealthy one and serves no one, least of all society as a whole. Perhaps this is further exacerbated by the terms 'conventional' and 'complementary' themselves, which do not clearly potray how they are often utilised in a very proactive and preventive way. In contrast, the conventional approach to healthcare is traditionally, at least financially speaking, reactive with the largest public health spending directed towards the smallest percentage of patients – those who are most seriously ill. This approach dictates that even countries with massive healthcare spending are no healthier than other countries that spend less. While this ensures the prolonged survival of the most ill, at the same time it reduces the amount that is available for spending on maintenance of health, or even prevention of ill health.

These days, some Western-based conventional medical practitioners, who largely began with the paradigm of technology and the treatment of the body in isolation, often incorporate aspects of the more 'Eastern' approach through acupuncture, acupressure, shiatsu, aromatherapy, ayurvedic massage, reflexology and Reiki. Interestingly, and when considering medicine in terms of what we know of the brain and how it works (see Part II), the more modern Western approach has emphasised developments based on language, logical analysis and a linear development of understanding, and can be seen to be based on the work of the left hemisphere of the brain. By contrast, the more Eastern cultures refined an approach based on imagery and a more holistic understanding, and developed largely based on intuition. This can be associated with the work of the right hemisphere of the brain.

In my opinion, the term 'complementary and alternative medicine' (CAM) is actually misleading and only really makes sense if used solely from the standpoint of Western medical practices. If a method or therapy works, it is neither complementary nor alternative. However, I suppose that in this context 'complementary' could also suggest that the approach may complement the body's own resources, and in so doing provide any extra help that the body may need at the time of poor health.

Anyone on a stroke prevention programme who suffers from hypertension should be aware that many doctors and psychologists are now studying the branch of science called psychoneuroimmunology (PNI), which concerns the interaction of emotions, the brain and immune systems. PNI has identified that our emotions play an important role in our physical health. For example, it is evident that stress depresses the immune system and can delay the production of antibodies, and that emotions associated with feelings of helplessness (commonplace in modern living!) or coping with bereavement can in fact lower an individual's resistance to illness.

It is important to realise that these factors will not automatically create organic disorders – nothing is as functionally simple as that. Lifestyle influences, such as demonstrating a life-long commitment to maintaining good health, feeling invigorated by life's challenges, or finding meaning in life (e.g. through religious faith), can reduce the risk of 'stress-related' disease. As a result, PNI researchers now use phrases such as 'the biology of belief', because as the mind can cause illness it can also help to overcome illness. This is where visualisation practice, hypnotherapy and certain other CAM treatments can be of value.

Nevertheless, I think it is worth mentioning that empirical studies into many CAM treatments are in their infancy and some therapists commit a pragmatic fallacy in simply stating that their treatment 'simply works' (Carroll 2003). Such comments are often made due to testimonial evidence from satisfied clients, with nobody keeping an accurate record of the failures, and they are therefore scientifically unsubstantiated. Any claims of positive results could equally be due to mood change of the patient, the placebo effect, natural regression (in that pain can come and go), the fact that pain itself is a subjective feeling, the fact that the body is naturally good at repairing itself, and that employing such treatments often coincides with many simultaneous lifestyle changes.

With this in mind, I feel that society needs to try to ensure that emotionally and physically vulnerable and sick individuals do not self-diagnose and that they only seek treatment from appropriately qualified and endorsed therapists, or it is perfectly feasible that more harm than good could be the result. Personally, I consulted my doctors regarding everything that I introduced into my recovery plan. Of course, an individual or carer can do their own research by all means, but they should ensure that the CAM practitioner must have all the relevant credentials, insurance and licences required and that any treatment subsequently undertaken must supplement and not interfere with conventional treatment. Combining alternative treatments must also be considered carefully and each treatment should be evaluated on its own merit. If you have a burning desire to combine different treatments in an attempt to get better fast, it's always a good idea to seek advice first from the supervisory conventional medical practitioner. To this end, the various Stroke Associations that exist in countries around the world (refer to Appendix II) should be reliable sources of information, and in this way the helpful rather than the harmful can be considered, discarded or employed.

What role does conventional medicine play?

Surgical intervention, drug therapies and the application of scientific research as required remain of paramount importance to many stroke survivors and those at high risk of suffering a stroke. Some of the most recent and current developments include:

- a diagnostic device, known as 'Alladin', to diagnose the precise state of a stroke victim and so determine the correct treatment at every stage from initial assessment to recovery

- continued research into the initial assessment of patients presented with stroke symptoms

- the stretching of a narrowed artery with a balloon, known as percutaneous transluminal angioplasty

- the study of genetic 'markers' that may identify those at risk of stroke may be used to predict atrial fibrillation, congestive heart failure, and atherosclerosis

- the injection of gas-filled bubbles into the bloodstream to burst blood clots

- the development of leg implants, known as Stimustep, which can aid walking in stroke survivors by stimulating the nerves and muscles responsible for lifting and raising the foot

- the development of medication, known as rimonabant, to help obese individuals to lose weight

- the cutting of salt levels in food

- continued research into the possible benefits of injecting testosterone into male stroke victims

- research into natural ways of reducing LDL (bad) cholesterol (e.g. research into the benefits of rice and vitamin E)

- continued research worldwide into secondary disease problems

- the continued research worldwide into rehabilitation programmes.

Despite the necessary application of resources to researching and developing these medical advances, I believe that the role of lifestyle changes and some additional players should not be downplayed. This opinion is shared by many doctors who know that, far from diminishing the significance of such breakthroughs, the potential impact of lifestyle changes, which are by nature very low-risk (as opposed to drugs, which have side-effects, and surgery, which has obvious dangers), will significantly reduce their need to get so involved in the healing process.

Among its targets, the Stroke Association (UK) is calling for:

- mandatory, consistent and clear labelling of food products

- a mandatory warning to be applied to food packaging when food contains more than a third (i.e. 2 grams) of the recommended amount of daily salt consumption

- mandatory, consistent and clear labelling of alcoholic drinks (especially in regard to the number of units)

- restrictions on junk food advertising (especially when aimed at children)

- a complete ban on smoking in all public places

- an increase in ring-fenced funding for stroke research.

We obviously cannot influence age or gender, but we can influence some of our unique individual health contributors. This is why the 'players to the game' approach as applied to healthcare can be so effective. It allows for a person's individual preferences, viewpoints and resources to be taken into account.

Player profiles

'It is common sense to take a method and try it. If it fails, admit it frankly and try another. Above all, try something.'

Franklin D. Roosevelt

What follows now are the players to the game, medical and non-medical, CAM and conventional. Many of these (marked with a star) I employed to aid my recovery from stroke; the remainder are additional, relevant players that other stroke survivors might use. However, due to the individual nature of stroke, I make no claims that this is an exhaustive list for stroke victims, survivors and carers. In terms of this book, the details of *players* are not nearly as important as the underlying *principles* that define the whole concept. In this way, the 'players to the game' approach to recovery and prevention can indeed be tailored to suit anyone – stroke survivors, relatives and carers can devise their own 'teams'.

I had been at home from hospital for some weeks re-orientating myself before I started with the basics. Rest became a player; nutrition became a player; walking became a player; quality time with Anne became a player; and strategies for coping emotionally with what had happened were each players.

As the months passed by, each of the following became additional players: my knowledge of anatomy and physiology; my understanding of chikung (simple energy exercises as associated with the Chinese interpretation of energy); my knowledge and application of acupressure (derived from traditional Chinese medicine, this is a form of treatment that involves pressure on particular points in the body known as 'acupressure points'); the use of visualisation; swimming; enlisting the help of CAM therapists; attending sports massage therapy; increasing my understanding about stroke; and writing this book (of course!).

As a result of my experience, I certainly agree with many doctors who believe that knowledge and motivation to get really involved in the healing process is more important than all the technology available in today's medicine. I have made it clear in earlier sections of the book that the consequences of my stroke left me having to focus primarily on aspects of movement, along with dealing psychologically with such a traumatic and major life event. Had it been necessary for me to attend a stroke club, such as a Dysphasia Group, that too would have been incorporated into my programme as a player. When I analysed the players, it became obvious that some could be further divided into distinct, individual players. For example, nutrition as one player should be divided into macronutrients, micronutrients, and even cooking methods – each of which needed to become a player to the game in its own right in order to develop a useful understanding of the role of each.

Please keep in mind that these players are simply listed and identified in alphabetical order, not in any order of priority.

Acupuncture and acupressure*

I have placed these together because they are so similar. Both are thought to have been practised in China for over 4000 years, and both rely on theories of traditional Chinese medicine (TCM) where specific points on the body (known as acu-points) are stimulated, either by needles or manual pressure, in order to regulate energy flow and encourage the body to heal itself. While most of the evidence regarding this is anecdotal, there is some scientific evidence to support that they contribute effectively to the management of pain – which can be a complication of stroke. My knowledge of acu-theory is detailed, and in fact my martial art teaching qualifications include a system that integrates these same points to disrupt energy flow and in so doing gain a real advantage over an assailant. I have absolutely no doubt as to the effectiveness of manipulating and stimulating the points on the body identified in traditional Chinese medicine. Furthermore, applying pressure to easily accessible acu-points is a good home treatment. As I had been advised against any neck massage due to the vertebral arterial dissection, which is the likely cause of my stroke, I utilised acu-points (located on the shoulders and even on the hands and feet) to help ease aches and tension in this area.

Anatomical position (understanding)*

The anatomical position is a position used as a reference when describing parts of the body in relation to each other. Used in conjunction with terms of movement, the anatomical position allows a standard way of documenting where one part of the body is in relation to another, regardless of whether the body is standing, lying down, or in any other position. In terms of stroke rehabilitation, physiotherapy, or exercising for prevention, understanding the anatomical position as a starting point for activity allows for clear descriptive instructions of certain exercises. In addition, simply lying in the anatomical position, with the back, shoulders and head supported with towels, is an excellent way of encouraging correct breathing.

When in the anatomical position, the body is not in the usual position adopted at rest. A person in the anatomical position is standing erect, eyes looking straight ahead, arms by the sides and the palms of the hands and toes directed forward.

Angioplasty and stenting

This is a surgical technique that is occasionally used to open the narrow part of an artery and so increase blood flow through the artery.

Anticoagulant drugs

Anticoagulant drugs may be prescribed in order to thin the blood, rather than those antiplatelet drugs prescribed to block the clotting cells (platelets) in the blood.

Antiplatelet drugs

Dipyridamole is sometimes prescribed with aspirin. In individuals who cannot tolerate or are advised against taking aspirin, the antiplatelet drug clopidogrel may be issued.

Appendicular skeleton (understanding)*

This is the part of the skeleton that includes the pectoral girdle, the pelvic girdle and the upper and lower limbs. It is essentially those parts attached to the core (middle) of the skeleton and includes those parts we could actually survive without.

Understanding this is paramount to working on improving human movement, and I regard it as an important cognitive player to the game. An appreciation of this is necessary in order to consider the best use of other endothermic and exothermic players.

See also Core strength, Kinesiology and Posture.

Aromatherapy

Aromatherapy, a term coined by French chemist René-Maurice Gattefosse in the 1920s, uses oils extracted from plants to aid healing. These oils are either inhaled or applied to the skin as part of a massage. While many claims made by aromatherapists have not been proved scientifically, aromatherapy may help to achieve a state of relaxation when used in conjunction with other players. This state may, in turn, make the body responsive to other players.

Aspirin*

Aspirin is very often suggested or prescribed for those at risk and for stroke survivors, with the exception of those involved in a haemorrhagic stroke. This very effective little tablet, originally derived from willow, operates on different levels. Most importantly, it reduces the body's production of thromboxane, a natural contributor to the 'stickiness' of blood platelets, which leads to an improvement in blood flow and consequently a reduced risk of blood clotting. Blood is perhaps at its 'stickiest' first thing in the morning, so this would be the logical time to take the aspirin. In addition, taking aspirin can reduce some of the residual pain often experienced by a stroke survivor and reduce oedema (swelling), which may occur with therapy.

Aspirin is now even believed to help protect people against Alzheimer's disease; however, it is very important to follow the prescribed dose and instructions. More is definitely not better and, unless taken after eating, there is a risk of an irritation to the stomach lining. Generally, a daily dose is prescribed to people whose five-year risk of a heart attack or stroke is 3 per cent or more. At age 50, 80 per cent of men and 50 per cent of women are at this level of risk. This has led to a continuing debate by some leading medical experts on whether to promote an age threshold approach, such as an indiscriminate policy advising everyone over the age of 50 to take a daily dose of aspirin. Some believe that it could do more harm than good in respect of the risk of a major gastro-intestinal bleed at age 60.

Axial skeleton (understanding)*

This is the part of the skeleton that includes the skull and spinal column (with sternum and ribs), which we could certainly not function without. It is the axis around which the appendicular skeleton moves. Understanding this is paramount to working on improving human movement and, as with the appendicular skeleton, I regard it as an important cognitive player to the game.

See also Core strength, Kinesiology and Posture.

Ayurvedic medicine (understanding)*

I consider this to be a cognitive player to the game, in that it relates to an umbrella system of understanding on health issues. Established over 5000 years ago this is the traditional, and remains the principal, Indian medicine. Like TCM, it focuses on preventing illness and maintaining good health through balancing mind, body and spirit. An imbalance will lead to ill health, which should be redressed with the aid of lifestyle changes that include attention to nutrition, yoga, meditation, visualisation, massage and herbal remedies.

Breathing*

Breathing can be both a conscious and unconscious physiological activity. When the body is experiencing a state of anxiety or stress, it prepares for a crisis. On such occasions, breathing occurs on a primary, unconscious level and the breathing rate (i.e. the number of breaths per minute) increases in an attempt to get more oxygen into the body. However, the lower lobes of the lungs, which are below the chest and normally inflate with little effort, are restricted by muscle tension in times of stress. To help compensate, the shoulders are lifted and the upper lobes of lungs are used. Meanwhile, heart rate and blood pressure increases in order to get oxygenated blood to the muscles. This is due in part to the fact that less than a tenth of a litre of blood flows through the top of our lungs every minute as opposed to the more than a litre of blood that flows through the bottom of the lungs each minute. To maintain the high rate of oxygen consumption, and to expel carbon dioxide, the breathing rate remains high, erratic and shallow. This impulsive inhalation and exhalation is called 'emergency breathing', or hyperventilation. Hyperventilation disturbs the body's blood pH balance (blood acidity), which prevents the oxygenated blood reaching the brain, organs and muscles. In addition, hyperventilating restricts the effective expulsion of many of the body's toxins – 70 per cent of which are expelled through our breath. Due to lifestyle and health issues, this breathing response can be triggered anywhere, and some people may actually spend most of the day in a state of hyperventilation. As you read this book you may even be hyperventilating.

The basic breathing techniques advocated in chikung practice (see below) aim to consciously help combat such restrictive breathing and have sound physiological support. A sleeping person, or a baby, illustrates a good way of breathing. Such deep, rhythmic breathing triggers a relaxation response, which is the opposite physiological response to the 'fight or flight' response we feel as a result of the cocktail of chemicals released in times of stress. This relaxation response can even be measured physiologically, and the signs are the exact opposite to those evident at times of stress. They include stimulation of the parasympathetic nervous system (see Glossary), which results in a slower heart rate and increased blood flow to the appendicular skeletal system (i.e. the extremities). This belly or diaphragm breathing lessens the stress reaction by 'short circuiting' the sympathetic nervous system (which responds to stress). So, by concentrating on relaxed, focused breathing, the blood pH stabilises and more oxygen can get to the brain, organs and muscles.

The target breathing rate should be around 12 breaths per minute, although this is generally much higher than it needs to be. At around 12 breaths per minute, heart rate and blood pressure drop automatically. This conscious attention to breathing can be undertaken lying, sitting, standing or moving and should help the body to rediscover its natural balance.

See also Chikung and Sympathetic nervous system.

Chikung*

Chikung is mentioned in many Chinese books, dating back hundreds of years. One such work, the *I Ching Book of Changes*, was written in 2852BC by a practitioner called Fu Xi. This work was later modified and developed by another practitioner, the ruler of the state of Zhou, Wen Wang, in 1122BC. A reasonable explanation of chikung is that it is the Chinese art of developing vital energy. In China, physicians sought to develop this energy for healing; *gongfu* (kung fu) exponents developed it for increasing combat efficiency; Confucian scholars developed it for mind expansion; and Taoist and Buddhist practitioners cultivated it for spiritual growth.

The many benefits associated with and attributed to the practice of chikung can be explained simply in Western terms. Through controlled breathing, physical movement and visualisation, an individual reaches a state where body and mind are simply working in harmony, in the way they are supposed to. The *chi* (energy) then provides the necessary information to all parts of the body and mind, so producing just the right types of chemicals of the right amounts at the right places at the right times. When all systems are functioning naturally, the Chinese figuratively describe this condition as that of a harmonious *chi* flow.

According to Chinese medical thought, practising chikung can help cure or control, as well as prevent, all kinds of illness including diseases like asthma, diabetes, hypertension and some psychological problems.

There are possibly thousands of types of chikung, with most methods having their own, individual levels of attainment for practitioners. I opted to practise a simple, very static, chikung set which is known as the 5-element Chikung Set.

See also Breathing and Visualisation.

Chiropractic manipulation

This is based on the theory put forward in the 19th century by an American grocer, Daniel Palmer. He proposed that misalignments of the spine (subluxations) are the cause of many medical problems and that the misalignments interfere with the nervous system and prevent the body from contributing to healing itself.

In terms of stroke, chiropractic manipulation must at times be viewed with great caution. My consultant advised me against any neck manipulation due to the possibility of a further vertebral arterial dissection. In many countries throughout the world there is a debate between various chiropractic organisations and the conventional medical profession about the risks of neck manipulation. It is important to repeat again that the advice of the conventional medical supervisor should be sought before employing additional treatment.

Commitment*

I have never been short of commitment to any given task, and with the passing of time after my stroke came to realise that it should not rob me of this quality. I have always demonstrated commitment, rather than natural ability, in almost all of my academic and physical endeavours. I consider myself fortunate in this regard. After all, commitment is not a definable skill that can be taught. Rather it is a transferable attitude. It can be applied to different tasks, or gently coaxed out of others. I am grateful that I have had a natural absolute belief that I would accomplish what I wanted to, or needed to, accomplish as I have gone through life.

I suppose an individual lacks commitment towards something when they do not care enough about it. In matters of health and quality of life, is it possible to care too much? After my stroke, I read a great deal that has been written about commitment, and while much of it was not written exclusively in the context of illness, the message was always the same. Your commitment should not waver even when your goal seems to be unreachable. Commitment is actually taking responsibility for yourself. Committed people are those that do not find excuses, but act in a manner consistent with the successful achievement of their goals.

Components of fitness (general) *

Fitness is not any one thing. I consider that fitness is made up of four key parts:

- physical fitness

- mental fitness

- social fitness

- emotional fitness.

Before my stroke I paid most attention to physical fitness. Post-stroke, my recovery and stroke prevention programme had to focus on each area. They each provided me with very distinct and identifiable challenges, and I met them all with various, and ever-changing, degrees of success.

Components of physical fitness *

Physical fitness is a blend of a number of physical qualities. The term 'physical fitness' is most often used to describe a person's physical condition, which is the result of differing fitness components working together in order to influence overall physical efficiency. It is generally accepted that physical fitness is made up of 11 different parts, of which five are classified as health-related and six are classified as skill-related.

Components of health-related fitness

1. Cardiovascular fitness – the ability to perform large muscle, dynamic, moderate to high-intensity exercise for long periods of time

2. Strength – the maximal force that can be generated by a specific muscle or muscle group

3. Endurance – the ability of a muscle group to perform repeated contractions (i.e. work) over a period of time

4. Flexibility – the ability to move a joint through a range of motions

5. Body composition – the relative ratio of fat to fat-free body mass (i.e. fat compared to bones and muscle).

Components of skill-related fitness

1. Agility – the ability to change the position of the body quickly and to control the movement of the whole body

2. Balance – the maintenance of a desired position

3. Co-ordination – the ability to use the eyes with one or more body parts

4. Power – the ability to quickly perform a movement involving strength

5. Reaction time – the amount of time it takes to move after seeing, hearing or feeling a stimulus

6. Speed – the ability to perform a movement quickly.

My physical training before the stroke had paid due attention to all of these components of physical fitness, and many had been developed to a very advanced level. However, my stroke rehabilitation and prevention programme considered these components at their most basic level. Consequently, I had to prioritise some to be the players requiring my most urgent and immediate attention. These were cardiovascular fitness (which, with nutrition as a complementary player, had a direct effect on body composition); flexibility (supported with sports massage therapy as its complementary player); balance (supported with core strength work as its complementary player); and co-ordination (supported with repetition of daily activities and core strength work as complementary players). In this way, redeveloping the components of physical fitness became intrinsically linked to almost all other players.

Core strength*

When someone talks about core strength, they are referring to all of the muscles deep within the abdominal area and back (attaching to the spine or pelvis), and in the pelvic area and hips. Many of the core muscles cannot be seen because they are buried underneath other muscles. Full details are not required in this book, but the core region includes the abdominals (rectus, transverse, and obliques), the back extensor muscles (erector spinae), and the side flexors (quadratus lumborum). Of importance to some stroke survivors will be the fact that the transverse abdominus (the deepest layer) is one of the primary respiratory muscles.

The core is important because it is where movement originates and it is the source of our stability. It is the muscles in the core that link the upper and lower body together, helping to co-ordinate movement and transmit forces from one part to another. In terms of sport, athletes that possess a strong core will be able to better manage the body's motions as they learn to perform at higher speeds. In terms of everyday movement, if the core muscles are weak then the body does not work effectively and other muscles have to compensate. This can result in poor control of the appendicular skeleton, postural problems and injuries such as a twisted ankle or knee, a pulled shoulder, or the classic 'bad back'. I suffered with all of these problems as a result of the cerebellar damage. Through a degree of ignorance on my part, it was actually a year after my stroke and six months after beginning swimming before I began working on core strength. I soon paid due attention to this player after a consultation with a new physiotherapist (in terms of my stroke), and I noticed improvements very quickly.

See also Homeostasis, Mirror therapy, Sports massage therapy and 'Swiss Ball' body rolling for core strength.

Counselling*

Nine months after my stroke, due to changes within my GP's medical centre, I started seeing a senior partner in the practice. He suggested that I make an appointment with the surgery's counsellor as the stroke had resulted in subsidiary worries in addition to my health, including ones related to financial matters and my career. I followed up on this and consequently had a series of sessions with the counsellor and later with a consultant psychiatrist. Due to the individual nature of stroke, this player may or may not be relevant to other stroke survivors.

Equipment

A variety of specialised equipment may be introduced and recommended to the individual/client/patient by the occupational therapist and physiotherapist for use by the stroke survivor in the short, medium or long term.

Essential oils*

Essential oils are volatile, oily, fragrant liquids extracted from plant leaves, bark, wood, stems, flowers, seeds, buds, roots, resins and petals. There are many uses for essential oils, from therapeutic baths to scented room sprays. Anne took charge of this and used geranium, lavender, lemon, lemongrass and ylang ylang for calming; added sandalwood to baths to reduce anxiety; and used ginger to encourage a feeling of energy. However, it is important to remember to be cautious about putting most essential oils on your skin, particularly citrus oils, as they are highly concentrated and can cause serious reactions.

Financial management*

In order to be able to apply oneself to a programme of recovery (rather than a programme of prevention) after stroke, financial worries have to be kept in context. However, this can be very difficult, even after such a harrowing experience. I had been very well advised by my independent financial adviser over a period of some years and I knew that I was well covered by a range of insurance and protection policies. Nevertheless, with almost 18 months of uncertainty about returning to teaching, financial worries emerged as one of the biggest, consistent problems I encountered after the stroke. However, if I had not been as well covered by policies as I was, things would have been a whole lot worse. See Chapter 11 for more information in this area.

FITT guidelines*

The FITT guidelines should be considered in conjunction with all forms of therapy and will be useful for those stroke survivors who are able to become more independent in terms of how they can contribute to, and support, their recovery. Walking is something that many stroke survivors are able to resume to some extent, often independently, so by using this activity as an example, the usefulness of these guidelines will become clear.

- **Frequency** – How often? This is the number of times that a walk is taken a week. Research shows physiological improvements occur with three to five sessions per week. This is not to say that walking less frequently will be pointless, just that the benefits will be less.

- **Intensity** – How hard? The general rule for anyone recovering from illness or injury is to take it easy. The less active a person is, or has been, the less it will take to give them a good workout. As the body gets used to walking, more effort can be put in.

- **Time** – How long? A worthwhile walk does not have to take hours. This is where the advice of the medical staff will be invaluable.

- **Type** – How appropriate? The type of activity should be considered carefully. For example, walking on a flat surface would be considered a different type of activity to walking up or down an incline.

See also Core strength, Goal setting and recognising achievement, Homeostasis, Kinesiology, Principles of training and Secondary prevention.

Goal setting and recognising achievement*

To help with this, I read personal accounts written by stroke victims, or stroke survivors. I researched different medical perspectives of the illness of stroke – including causes, treatments and effects. Inevitably, rather than this helping me to establish goals for myself, I became plagued with doubts about myself, and about the future. Consequently, I found it hard to set myself goals. I even did something that was alien to me until I had the stroke. I gave something up. I conceded defeat. I stopped writing. I concluded that my goal of writing this book was an irrational idea.

As the months went by I made a conscious decision to become disciplined with regard to positive thinking, and utilised the player of commitment. I realised that at the core of human behaviour is purpose. In other words, having a deeper value for how we live our lives. Purpose may be long-term, or short-term. These days, however, it is often confused with quality of life. I gradually moved through the process of denial and became able to face my fears, and recognise my progress with a new and enhanced value and appreciation of my life. Society places many pressures on inter-personal relationships, possessions, rewards at work, and the development of new skills. Sometimes, real purpose is lost to short-term desire. Now that I understand that, I believe I am now far closer to realising my individual potential. I began writing again as I discovered this new sense of purpose.

In the business world, it is often said that goals are those things you want, while outcomes are those things you create. I have found this to be true in my personal and professional life, as outcomes are even evident as a result of inaction. In such cases, however, the outcome does not normally match the goal. Setting a challenging, yet realistic, goal, and acting to ensure that the goal turns into the outcome, seems to be the key to remaining positive in the face of adversity. At times, additional support may be needed and so all goals should be considered from a wider viewpoint or different perspective when set. Otherwise, any failure may be branded a catastrophe. To avoid this, I suggest that, when you set yourself a series of goals, you should pick the easiest as your first target. Then application of a positive mindset must be both evident and consistent, and cannot be confined to being a Sunday morning activity. An important aspect of this whole process is recognising the achievements that are made. In this way, success can be enjoyed and the process is positively reinforced. New goals can then be set, and will not be limited by what is deemed to be currently possible.

See also Positive thinking and Visualisation.

Herbal medicine

Worldwide, this is the most widely used alternative medicine and is used by many cultures. Basically, thousands of plants have been used medicinally for thousands of years. In TCM, for example, the concept of 'herb' may be better translated as 'drug'.

Herbal remedies may be a mixture of one or more herbs and come in many forms including as raw herbs, capsules, tablets and ointments. In terms of stroke prevention, *Ginkgo biloba* is believed to reduce cholesterol, soften cerebral blood vessels and improve circulation; while *Ganoderma lucidum* is said to reduce blood viscosity. However, many herbs have not been subject to scientific study and some can be very potent. Obviously, in terms of stroke, anyone thinking about introducing herbal remedies should consult their supervising conventional doctor.

Homeostasis (understanding)*

Homeostasis is a fundamental characteristic of ecological, biological and social systems. In humans, it has a survival value as it means that if the equilibrium is unbalanced by some 'irritant', however large or small, then our biological system will attempt to evolve and not simply endure it.

In more simple terms, physical exercises under the guidance of therapists are designed to be a form of positive stress (i.e. irritants). When such positive stress is applied, the body temporarily moves into a state of alarm, and begins to make adaptations in an effort to regain its equilibrium. In grand terms, it may therefore be possible to adapt to a changing environment and so sustain life. As human biological systems are generally durable, they will actually grow stronger as a result of the stress, simply because the systems perceive that the stress will be encountered again.

Any physical improvements, or 'motor learning', that result from physical therapy are due to the process of homeostasis. However, if the stress is inappropriate, is too sudden or severe, then the biological systems will not be able to adapt and may be permanently damaged. The qualified therapist will be able to consider individual physical, psychological and emotional differences between stroke survivors and make recommendations appropriately. Appreciating homeostasis is a cognitive player to the game and can be seen on many levels, in many of the players discussed in this section.

Hydration*

A nutrient that is often overlooked is water. There are different rules of thumb regarding how much to drink, including 'eight glasses per day', or 'enough to keep your urine clear and odourless', and 'just calculate the ounces of water to drink each day by taking your body weight in pounds and divide that number in half'. How much an individual needs really depends on many factors, including their health status, activity levels and even where they live. The simplest guide is to drink to prevent feelings of thirst, rather than to react to feelings of thirst. Generally, this does not happen and Western societies are full of chronically dehydrated individuals.

What is a more straightforward issue is why we must drink water. Water is crucial to health, and every system in the body depends on it. It is cholesterol-free, calory-free, fat-free, and low in sodium. Every day we lose water through sweating, expiration, and bladder and bowel emptying. Lack of water can lead to dehydration, which is when there is not enough water in the body to carry on normal functions. Even mild dehydration, with a loss of 1 per cent of body weight, results in a decrease in blood volume and can lead to head and vision problems and fatigue. The stroke survivor cannot afford to have any additional, and avoidable, discomfort in this way. Of course, individuals suffering additional conditions, such as those that impair water secretion, should limit their intake on the advice of medical practitioners.

Hydrotherapy

Hydrotherapy is the use of water in the treatment of disease, and hydrothermal therapy additionally uses its temperature effects, as in hot baths, saunas and wraps. Water therapy has been around for centuries, and both methods of treatment have been used for the treatment of disease and injury by many cultures, including those of ancient Greece, Rome, China and Japan. Water is an important ingredient in the traditional Native American healing systems.

The treatment increases circulation, contributes to general wellbeing and may help with pain control. A number of techniques are available under the general heading of hydrotherapy, including: baths and showers, neutral baths, sitz baths, contrast sitz baths, foot baths, cold mitten friction rub, steam inhalation, hot compresses, cold compresses, alternating hot and cold compresses, heating compresses, body wrap, wet sheet pack, and salt glow.

Kinesiology*

This is the branch of physiology that studies the mechanics and anatomy in relation to human movement. The quality of all movement is based on a kinetic chain – the subtle interaction of joints and muscle contraction, which determines our structural health. We should remember that if a human body were stripped of all tissue, the bones of the skeleton would fit together perfectly. It is the muscles and the system controlling them that distort movement, and there are endless varieties of movement problem patterns that can exist in just one body. The human body is subject to mechanical flaws as a result of injuries or disease (including stroke); the effects of gravity and ageing; not exercising, over exercising and performing the wrong type of exercise; poor posture; and psychological stress. However, we can re-adjust the body and so improve its structure and movement. I was fortunate to have followed a degree in human movement studies and to have had a long-standing interest in anatomy and physiology. Nevertheless, I still invested time in widening my knowledge after my stroke and consider this to have been a vital cognitive player to the game, which directly contributed to me implementing many players.

See also Core strength, Mirror therapy, Posture, Sports massage therapy and 'Swiss Ball' body rolling for core strength.

Macronutrients*

Macronutrients are protein, carbohydrates and fats. With the obvious exception of eating specifically for sports performance, there are many suggestions about the best ratio of macronutrients in the diet – the most common one being 50 per cent carbohydrate, 20 per cent protein and 30 per cent fat. For stroke survivors, an individual programme of intake should be prepared in consultation with a dietician. This will often be based on more than simply eating to survive and to paying attention to recommended daily amounts. However, what is important is the cumulative intake of meals, as opposed to individual foods, and that meals are eaten regularly, preferably every four hours. For individuals paying attention to lowering their cholesterol, this should include a complex carbohydrate, however small the amount, last thing at night.

Protein

Protein comes from the Greek word *protos*, meaning 'first'. It is used for energy, growth and repair and can be safely increased during periods of calorific restriction.

Carbohydrates

Carbohydrates provide an important source of energy, and the only source of dietary fibre, which is essential for good digestion and for lowering the glycemic index (GI) of foods (see Glossary). Carbohydrates are categorised as either monosaccharides (simple) or polysaccharides (complex), based on the type of sugar molecule and consequently the speed with which the body breaks it down. Simple carbohydrates include sugars such as glucose, sucrose, fructose and dextrose; they have a high GI and so enter the bloodstream quickly. Complex carbohydrates are found in grains, vegetables and some fruits; they have a low GI and so cause a slow steady rise in blood sugar.

Fats

Fats can generally be classified as either saturated (i.e. solid at room temperature) or unsaturated (i.e. liquid at room temperature). Unsaturated fats can be further classified as polyunsaturated and monounsaturated (see Table 10.1). The Seven Countries Study (Keys 1970) conducted between 1958 and 1970 illustrated a link between saturated fat and heart disease. Saturated fat intake should be kept low and monitored very carefully, but it should be known that an inadequate amount of unsaturated fat may also adversely affect health by lowering LDL (the 'good') cholesterol. The problem in many developed countries is that while total fat intake has remained unchanged in recent years, the relative proportion of saturated fats (also found in highly processed convenience foods) consumed has increased dramatically. This has undoubtedly helped to accelerate the increase of heart disease and stroke in those countries. Olive and rapeseed (canola) oil, which contains mainly monounsaturated fat, lowers total and LDL cholesterol without decreasing HDL cholesterol when used instead of saturated fat.

Table 10.1 The classification of fats and their effect on cholesterol

Type of fat	Examples of food source	Effect on cholesterol
Saturated fat	Full-cream dairy products and palm oil used in convenience/pre-packed/take-away foods	Raises
Trans fat	Dairy products, some meats, and many commercially prepared foods	Raises
Polyunsaturated fat	Vegetable oils, some margarines, vegetables and fish oil	Lowers
Monounsaturated fat	Olive, rapeseed and peanut oil, avocados and nuts	Lowers

Fibre

Dietary fibre is the general term for the indigestible part of fruits and vegetables. Fibre is not an energy source but aids digestion and protects the health of your colon; and increasingly, certain types of plant fibres are being found to have other beneficial roles in maintaining health. Increasing the amount of fibre in your diet has numerous health benefits. Fibre can be either soluble (i.e. able to dissolve in water) or insoluble. Soluble fibre can lower cholesterol, while insoluble fibre can prevent bowel problems. An intake of 25 to 30g per day is thought essential for maintaining health.

Sources of soluble fibre	Sources of insoluble fibre
Oats (bran, cereals and breads)	Wholegrain (pasta, bread and cereal)
Beans (chickpeas, lentils, soya and baked beans)	Brown rice
Some fruits (strawberries and citrus)	Fruit and vegetables

Massage therapy*

Massage therapy is claimed to benefit all people. There is a great variety, in terms of types of massage therapy available, with many originating in exotic parts of the world. Some use a combination of techniques in order to achieve the desired effect, such as oils, music, friction and pressure; while others are complex mixtures of holistic healing practices involving physical, emotional and spiritual components.

I opted for sports massage therapy (not to be confused with a relaxing massage!), which I consider to have been an extremely effective player to the game.

See also Core strength, Homeostasis, Mirror therapy and Posture.

Media reports*

It is very important to keep media stories in context, in terms of who is reporting information and why they are reporting it. However, I consider keeping abreast of new research and ideas an important player. To be honest, since I have been paying particular attention to matters relating to the illness of stroke, rarely has a week gone by without me finding an article associated with stroke. These include ones relating to headings such as 'Binge drinkers double risk of having a stroke warn doctors', 'Men warned of stroke risk from three alcoholic drinks a day', 'High levels of homocysteine may increase risk of stroke', 'Sudden neck movement and cervical artery dissection', 'Testosterone boosts recovery from strokes', 'Call for more stroke units', 'Statins cause wrinkles', 'Eating kiwi fruits could prevent strokes' and 'Salt and stroke'.

Micronutrients*

Micronutrients are vitamins and minerals and are essential for life. They are distinct from macronutrients in that they are only required in tiny amounts. They are often available in supplement form, the provision of which is a multi-billion dollar industry. For example, women may benefit from a calcium or iron supplement; older individuals may benefit from a vitamin B12 supplement; and vegans may need vitamins D, B12 and riboflavin. The need for any additional supplementation should be discussed with a nutritionist. While many doctors contend that we can get all that we need from our food, and that the benefits of supplements occurs only when they are taken as part of a healthy eating pattern, some surveys show that many people, even in developed countries (e.g. the US), consume less than two thirds of the recommended daily allowance of micronutrients.

Fish oils

I found out that fish oils are good for brain development as well as joints, circulation and heart function. The brain uses approximately 25 per cent of all the energy produced by the body, and I wanted to ensure that my brain was given all the energy it needs. Similarly, a great deal of the brain's energy is devoted to the body. I decided I wanted to give my brain and body every opportunity of working collaboratively and effectively. Anne and I started to eat more fresh fish and I sought to get the essential ingredients for health from food. Oily fish is the richest source of the polyunsaturated fatty acids eicosapentaenoic (EPA) and docosahexaenoic (DHA), or omega-3 fatty acids. Omega-3 can contribute to the lowering of high blood pressure; it can help reduce inflammatory problems such as arthritis, which cause pain; and it can make blood less sticky and less likely to form blood clots where clots are not wanted. The Fish Foundation publicises the fact that, for the elderly, omega-3 can reduce the risk of death from heart attack and stroke if combined with other strategies. I opted to supplement my food intake with 1g per day of cod liver oil tablets containing added omega-3 fatty acids, as they can be hard to get from a normal diet.

Fish sources of omega-3	Plant sources of omega-3
Mackerel	Flaxseed and flaxseed oil
Trout	Walnuts and walnut oil
Salmon	Sweet potatoes and pumpkins

Co-enzyme Q10

I also began to take co-enzyme Q10 (CoQ10), something I took daily when I was actively competing in sport. CoQ10 plays an important role in the process of converting food nutrients into the energy that cells need, particularly the cardiac cells of the heart, in order to function. This vital supplement may be of particular importance to those of us that take cholesterol-lowering statin drugs (statins). As we get older, the body makes less CoQ10, and what it does make can be dramatically depleted by statins. In Canada, for example, every packet of statins warns of CoQ10 depletion.

Vitamins

I increased my intake of vitamins C and E with fresh vegetables and fruit. Fruit and vegetables are not only high in vitamins and minerals, but also in the nutrient antioxidants, which prevent free-radical toxins from causing LDLs to contribute to artery lining and so cause atherosclerosis. Free-radical toxins are produced naturally in the body, but in excess they modify the LDLs, making them 'bad'. Antioxidants prevent them from getting out of control and causing damage to cell membranes.

Garlic

I added more garlic to food, which over a period of years can reduce cholesterol and reduce the risk of thrombosis.

Glucosamine and chondroitin sulphate

I had been taking a daily supplement of glucosamine sulphate with chondroitin for some years and decided to maintain this after the stroke. Glucosamine is classified as an amino sugar, which, unlike other sugars, are carbohydrates incorporated into body tissue rather than being used as an energy source. As such, glucosamine is involved in the formation of cartilage, ligaments, tendons, bones, eyes, nails and heart valves. Chondroitin sulphate is part of a large protein molecule (proteoglycan) that gives cartilage elasticity.

Mirror therapy*

Mirror therapy has been employed with good effect with stroke survivors suffering from hemiparesis (Altschuler *et al.* 1999). Mirror therapy involves patients trying to move their hands or arms symmetrically, while all the time watching the movement of the good arm in a mirror. In such cases, it provides patients with proper visual input because the reflection helps the patient think that their affected arm is moving correctly, even though it may not be, hence stimulating the brain to help with the nerve control required for limb movement.

I did not have hemiparesis, but I did have some co-ordination, postural, balance and gait problems. Looking at my reflection, I was surprised at how badly my body lacked the symmetry it had before the stroke. I incorporated mirror therapy into my daily routine for some months, and this combined with massage therapy and core strength work resulted in real and visible improvements in these areas.

See also Core strength, Goal setting and recognising achievement, Kinesiology, Positive thinking, Posture, Sports massage therapy and Visualisation.

Nutrition*

All biological systems need a supply of energy. This energy is derived from the nutrients eaten and through the chemical and biological processes of the digestive system. As I have said above, all nutrients are classified as either macronutrients, which are sources of calories, or micronutrients, which are vital in ensuring that the body makes better use of the macronutrients (see also Macronutrients and Micronutrients).

Those individuals seeking to prevent stroke, as well as stroke survivors, will probably encounter the term 'energy balance' at some point. Metabolic energy is measured in calories, and the energy balance is simply when the calories taken into the body equal the calories expended.

Energy balance: calories in = calories out

The average person needs an intake of 2600 calories per day to keep the energy balance. Individuals trying to prevent stroke may include weight loss as an aim of their preventive programme. Such people will need either to reduce their intake of calories or increase their output of calories. Stroke survivors, in the short term, may not require 2600 calories per day and be unable to increase their output of calories. They may, therefore, need to reduce their intake of calories accordingly.

With the aid of a variety of healthy eating and low-fat cook books, Anne and I now eat nicer, fresher food than before, which takes the same amount of time to prepare as a microwave meal takes to cook from frozen. Four months to the day from having my stroke, I had an appointment with my consultant, Dr Shetty. At the 'weigh-in' I found that I had lost more than a stone in weight since the stroke. While some weight loss was obviously muscle, a significant amount was simply excess body weight. This had been achieved without the 'Atkins Diet' or any published dietary plan and without any aerobic exercise whatsoever at that time. It had been achieved through a personal refinement of the 'Nutrition' player, which suited my needs at that time. At 12st 6lbs, my 5ft 11in frame was only 2lb in excess of the 12st 4lbs I had naturally maintained for about ten years between the ages of 18 and 28. Significantly, my cholesterol level had dropped from 6.4 mg/dl to 3.4 mg/dl in three months. This was good, because medical practitioners advocate keeping cholesterol levels below 5 mg/dl. According to the information given to me by the British Heart Foundation, only 20 per cent of this reduction could be attributed to the simvastatin. It is clear, therefore, that I was directly responsible for the rest of the reduction.

Occupational therapy*

Occupational therapy (OT) involves exercise and training to help the stroke patient relearn everyday activities such as eating, drinking and swallowing, dressing, bathing, cooking, reading and writing, and using the toilet. The goal of OT is to help the patient become independent or semi-independent. The therapist will work with an individual, paying attention to individual requirements, and may suggest the use of equipment ranging from wheelchairs to cutlery. I received an occupational assessment, rather than OT, when in hospital. At home, I suppose I took charge of my own OT.

Osteopathy

Osteopathy is credited to Dr Andrew Still, a US Civil War Union Army surgeon. As with chiropractic manipulation, osteopathy claims that realigning the body through manual manipulation encourages the body to heal itself. Again, neck manipulation can be a risk factor for stroke, and the advice of the conventional medical supervisor should be sought before employing additional treatment.

Parasympathetic nervous system (understanding)*

The parasympathetic nervous system is one of the two divisions of the autonomic nervous system (the other being the sympathetic nervous system). It consists of nerve fibres that leave the brainstem and sacral (lower) portion of the spinal cord and extend to nerve cell clusters (ganglia) at specific sites. In general, the parasympathetic nervous system opposes physiological effects of the sympathetic nervous system and is involved with the conservation of energy. It slows down the heart rate, constricts the pupils, stimulates digestive secretions, and dilates blood vessels.

Understanding this physiological system is a cognitive player to the game and will enhance many of the other players.

See also Sympathetic nervous system.

Positive thinking*

It seemed to me, in the months after my stroke, that the term 'stroke victim' by definition was a negative one. On the other hand, the term 'stroke survivor', by definition, is a positive one. This was the seed from which I tried to develop a positive mental attitude.

There are no magic steps to having a positive mental attitude. In my experience, even the most positive among us are prone to negative thinking. The key, if there is one, is to look for the good and positive, while becoming disciplined about what you say and think. In terms of stroke, the bad is an obvious source of mental focus, but every effort should be made to take a break from it, for however short a time this may be possible, in order to prevent it from being the only source of mental focus. Serious illness is unfair, and stroke survivors should not make the worst out of their situation because they feel hard done by. This, I know, is easy to say, but the emotional turmoil and response is really quite unpredictable.

I quickly accepted that other people had suffered more serious physical and cognitive effects following their stroke than I had with mine. However, instead of celebrating the fact that I was starting to recover I gradually started to feel an emotion similar to guilt, in that my stroke was not as bad as it could have been. At times, this emotion became very strong, but I was so embarrassed about thinking this way I did not dare mention it to anyone. Why had it not been as bad for me as it had been for other people? I know now that a state of confusion and exaggerated conflict of emotions had become the norm of my daily life since being admitted to hospital and I was just learning to live with some extremes. A stroke brings with it insecurities and uncertainty, and I cannot adequately portray what a shattering blow to my confidence having, and even surviving, the stroke actually was.

Nevertheless, throughout the months that followed my stroke, I never found myself asking the question 'Why me?' This would have wasted time and energy – both of which I intended to preserve fully. Rather, I repeatedly asked questions of myself: Who am I now, really? Where am I now in my life? Why did this happen to me now? What can I learn from this now? Where can I go next from here? As the well-known saying goes, 'Life is not a race, but a journey to be savoured each step of the way. Yesterday is history, tomorrow's a mystery and today is a gift. That's why we call it the present.'

It may be worth remembering that we often notice the change in others before they see it in themselves. Therefore, it is our friends and family who spot the signs that we are changing often before we do. With this in mind, we should perhaps always try to communicate effectively with those close to us.

See also Goal setting and recognising achievement and Visualisation.

Posture*

Posture implies being in a static state, whether standing, sitting or lying. However, this term is generally misunderstood – the human body is never completely static. Even the act of breathing involves various parts of the human structure moving in relation to one another. Almost without exception, and irrespective of whether someone has survived a stroke or not, we all have postural defects causing fragmentations in the rhythmically harmonious act of maintaining posture. For most individuals, even the simple act of maintaining proper posture causes muscle fatigue.

My posture suffered badly as a result of my stroke. The left side of my appendicular skeleton became very visibly different to the right side. Understanding the main issues relating to posture and redressing postural defects became a very important player.

See also Appendicular skeleton, Axial skeleton, Core strength, Kinesiology, Mirror therapy, Sports massage therapy and 'Swiss Ball' body rolling for core strength.

Power napping*

Stroke survivors inevitably become exhausted after comparatively little effort. For some, this will be a passing phase, confined to the initial months of recovery, while for others it will be long-lasting. Personally, I found it difficult to power nap regularly at times of tiredness so I would simply sit still and listen to quiet music. Those who can power nap may find it useful to adopt the approach of Thomas Edison and Salvador Dali, who apparently napped while holding a spoon or other unbreakable object. When they had been sleeping long enough or deep enough to cause the object to drop to the floor, waking them up, they would use the noise as a cue to get up feeling refreshed.

Prayer*

In difficult times, for example when dealing with the tragedy of stroke, some religious people lose their faith. This is, in fact, the time when they need it the most – after all, this is the essence of faith. Where there is suffering there will almost certainly be a religious response with people reaching out for support. All of us, regardless of religion or race, have to meet tragedy, disease and death. Prayer and meditation are tools frequently used by people the world over as they try to come to terms with sadness and illness. Some people certainly receive great strength from prayer whether they themselves are ill or they are grieving for someone else.

In my mind, prayer is not a restrictive concept and is certainly of little use if used only in times of hardship. I generally like to contemplate the words of others. One of my favourites was actually written by Anne, who has frequently produced simple, yet poignant prayers for school assemblies:

> Lord, we thank you for your love, For your protection from above, We know that you are always there, And that for each of us you care, You give us strength to carry on, Although the journey's hard and long, You give us all the minds to know, How to act, which way to go, Help us to use our minds and heart, To finish well the work we start, To choose to listen, when we should, To turn from evil and choose good, Thank you for the gifts you give, To help enrich the lives we live, In the days and weeks ahead, May we all by you be led, To work our hardest, try our best, And with a pinch of luck, be blessed.

Principles of training*

For a recovery or preventive programme to be effective it must be adjusted over time as the individual improves. The following principles (acronym SPORT) are important when planning or changing a programme, and are especially relevant to the physical aspects of such a programme:

- *Specificity* – This simply means that the muscles, energy systems or skills that are the focus for the intended improvement are the ones that should be challenged. For example, walking should contribute cardiovascular fitness while 'Swiss Ball' training will contribute to core strength.

- *Progression* – This is linked to the overload principle. As the body adapts to the therapy, the therapy should be made harder by any of the overload methods outlined below.

- *Overload* – This is the key to improving fitness. For fitness to improve, the body must work above its everyday level. This can be achieved by adapting the FITT guidelines:
    - ° **Frequency** – therapy may be taken more often
    - ° **Intensity** – therapy may be made harder than normal
    - ° **Time** – therapy sessions may last longer than normal
    - ° **Type** – therapy may alter.

- *Reversibility* – Some aspects of physical fitness are reversible. While stroke survivors may regain physical fitness up to a point, those seeking to prevent a stroke by undertaking an exercise programme should remember that it takes only three to four weeks for the body to lose the benefits of exercise, and for fitness levels to revert to what they were before the training programme was started.

- *Type* – The activity should be appropriate for the individual and may or may not involve, for example, an aid, staircase or hill.

Prozac

As the most popular antidepressant in the world, Prozac undoubtedly works and is reported not to be addictive. It may be introduced as a player by doctors, particularly in the case of an older stroke survivor.

Reflexology*

Apparently based on therapies used by ancient Egyptians, native Americans and the ancient Chinese cultures, reflexology involves manipulation of specific reflex areas in the foot, hands and ears that correspond to other parts of the body. Sometimes referred to as zone therapy, this therapy involves the application of pressure to these reflex zones in order to stimulate body organs and relieve areas of congestion. Similar to the principles of acupressure, reflexology works with the body's energy flow to stimulate self-healing and maintain a balance in physical function. The term 'reflexology' was introduced by an American, Eunice Ingham, in the early 1900s, and today reflexology is used to reduce pain, increase relaxation and stimulate circulation of blood and lymphatic fluids. It is perhaps especially useful in stress-related illness. Reflexology is also convenient in cases where an area of the body is traumatised or diseased to the extent that direct manipulation is not appropriate.

Relaxation*

> 'The more tranquil a man becomes, the greater his success, his influence, his power for good. Calmness of the mind is one of the most beautiful jewels of wisdom.'

James Allen (1864–1912), theologian and author

Relaxing should not be confused with laziness, or loafing about. It is being in a state, which can be still or moving, that is free from tension. A person can be relaxed and alert at the same time. The pace of modern-day living can affect the ability to relax as part of a stroke prevention programme, as can surviving a stroke (at least in the short term). It is perhaps at such times that we need to find the time to relax the most. An anxious mind cannot exist within a relaxed body (Jacobson 1974). I tried to remember this phrase as I began my daily recovery routine.

Dedicating part of the day to relaxation may prove an effective player for some people. For others, occasionally undertaking a body awareness review (BAR) may be a more suitable player. Most of us need to learn how to relax! At times of stress breathing may be erratic, shoulders may be raised and tight, hands may be clenched and teeth may grind. BAR can be undertaken whenever appropriate to check for the need to relax. It simply involves evaluating the level of anxiety and, if appropriate, initiating a response to counteract the tension. This may include some visualisation, stretching, and adjusting breathing and/or posture to reduce the tension. These relaxation checks and techniques are very pro-active and can be personalised to suit an individual's needs. We should not be afraid to treat ourselves to relaxation!

See also Breathing, Chikung, Secondary prevention, Sports massage therapy and Traditional Chinese medicine.

Secondary prevention*

This includes taking preventive measures after an individual has survived a stroke (as in my case) but, of course, applies equally to people who have had a transient ischaemic attack (see Glossary). For some people, secondary prevention will be quite straightforward. For others, this will involve a huge change of lifestyle and may result in changes to habits such as smoking, consumption of alcohol, participation in exercise, the management of stress, and the taking of drugs (including oral contraceptives and 'recreational' drugs). In certain cases, secondary prevention may involve surgery, but in all cases it should include becoming more knowledgeable about stroke. I include writing this book as a secondary prevention cognitive player to the game.

Self-hypnosis*

I opted to study hypnotherapy seriously in order to extend my use of visualisation. As I mentioned earlier, rather than just read a book and have a go, I enrolled to train as a clinical hypnotherapist with the BST Foundation at a prestigious London venue. As well as training to work with other people in a professional capacity, I also learnt to help myself. There are many misconceptions surrounding the science of hypnotherapy, largely due to the use of hypnosis in the field of entertainment. When encouraged to explore hypnotherapy from a medical perspective, it becomes clear that this naturally occurring phenomenon is an extremely powerful player. Part of the professional hypnotherapist's role should be to teach the client appropriate self-hypnosis techniques, and this is one of the questions that could be asked of a hypnotherapist when deciding whether or not to use one.

When learnt, self-hypnosis requires no assistance and no special environment. It activates a creative mind and helps to develop a positive state of mind and body. The result is that beliefs and action allow learning to occur. For many stroke survivors, the learned skill of self-hypnosis could undoubtedly be very beneficial, as an individual can, at a deep unconscious level, overcome some very limiting beliefs that may be present as a result of the stroke, be reminded of how the brain is able to learn, and begin to see themselves as much more than the person who has had a stroke.

See also Breathing, Chikung, Goal setting and recognising achievement, Kinesiology, Positive thinking, Posture, Traditional Chinese medicine and Visualisation.

Simplify life*

The same day that I was told that I had had a stroke, and while I was still confined to bed, I had an overwhelming feeling that I needed to simplify my life in the short and medium term. Given my previous active and ridiculously hectic daily routine, when the time came I found this surprisingly easy. Of course, I was very tired and confused for many weeks after the stroke, but even so, I knew instinctively that this was one of the most important players that I should pay attention to. Importantly, I learned to say 'no' to others, and 'yes' to myself and loved ones. This player, when linked to the 'Relaxation' player, allowed me to concentrate on surviving the event and getting better.

Good health, for most, seems to be a birthright, having been born fit, healthy and full of vitality. Too many of us lose our natural birthright along the way. For some this is due to circumstances beyond their control. For others, it is undoubtedly due to a careless disregard towards a state of wellbeing. Naturally, many people fall somewhere in between. I have been forced to contemplate reaching middle age rather than have the luxury of simply reaching and passing through it without any thought. If life is anything like a two-week holiday, then the second half passes by a lot faster than the first! I am determined to live what I hope will be at least the last half of my life on my terms, and I actually now feel better connected to the world around me and to society as a whole.

Simvastatin

Simvastatin is a drug used to reduce the amount of cholesterol and certain fatty substances in the blood. For more information see page 78.

Speech therapy

Speech therapy is a service provided by a healthcare professional that helps a person improve his or her ability to communicate. This includes both speech, which is how sounds are made, and language, which involves understanding and choosing the correct words to use. Speech problems, such as the inability to formulate coherent sentences or to understand verbal statements, are collectively known as aphasia. According to the National Aphasia Association, approximately 1 million Americans suffer from the condition, most of whom developed aphasia after a stroke. Some people will have swallowing problems as well as speech deficits. All these things can be addressed with the help of a speech therapist. Specific goals will be identified for each person, depending on which of the problems need to be improved.

Sports massage therapy*

Sports massage therapy (SMT) is a system of massage techniques aimed at maximising the potential of athletes to compete or perform. The practitioner sets out to identify key areas of the body that may need specific attention to release the potential of the muscle. This may include decongestion of a muscle or part of a muscle, release of restriction or improvement in range of movement. It works by utilising a range of massage techniques in a way that enhances the flow of congestion and waste products through the muscles and tendons. The SMT practitioner uses his or her skill to decide on which technique is best in which circumstances for the particular athlete concerned.

SMT has a different emphasis depending on which part of the athlete's training cycle they are in. The approach would be different in close season, pre-season and competition periods, the latter further specialised into pre-, intermediate and post-competition phases.

SMT also has many benefits with regard to injury prevention and recovery from injury although does not set out to treat injuries *per se*. In rehabilitation, SMT can help to stimulate the circulation, decongest muscles that may not have been used for months (depending on the situation) and to 'innovate' muscles or particular fibres to 'fire properly'. For example, if a leg is broken and is placed in a cast for months, once the cast has been removed, SMT can greatly assist the lymphatic system regain its circulation more quickly as the lymph system relies on movement of the muscles to aid circulation.

In the case of a stroke, there is no reason to assume that massage and other SMT techniques cannot assist in mobilising, stretching, decongesting and innovating muscles that have been directly affected by the stroke. Restoration of muscle control relies on stretch and strain, and it should be remembered that the muscles themselves have not been damaged by the stroke. In addition to the physiological benefits, there are also psychological benefits that can be experienced by the client enjoying deep tissue massage that can aid recovery.

See also Core strength, Kinesiology, Mirror therapy, Posture and 'Swiss Ball' body rolling for core strength.

St John's wort

Depression creeps up and affects over 50 per cent of stroke survivors. This is significant, as gross population statistics illustrate that this figure reduces to one in ten of the adult population. A 2005 German study concluded that St John's wort, when manufactured with the drug paroxine (aka Seroxat), is 'at least as effective in treating depression as a widely-prescribed antidepressant drug' and 'patients experienced fewer side effects' (Szegedi *et al.* 2005). The German researchers, who were financed by a company that markets the extract, have called for further related studies, but the conclusions will undoubtedly be noticed by the Medicines and Healthcare Regulatory Agency (MHRA), and the National Institute for Clinical Excellence (NICE), who only recently (December 2004) issued new guidelines on the use of drugs to treat depression.

In the meantime, it must be said that the British government has issued specific advice on the use of St John's wort. This includes advising individuals who are:

- taking treatment for migraine or depression who are also taking a St John's wort preparation to stop taking the St John's wort preparation as it may stop the medicine from working

- taking anti-convulsants for epilepsy or fits, theophylline for asthma or bronchitis, warfarin for blood clots, digoxin for heart condition, or cyclosporin following a transplant, who are also taking a St John's wort preparation, to stop taking the St John's wort preparation as it may stop the medicine from working properly (these individuals should see their pharmacist or doctor before doing so as the dose of the medicine may need to be altered to prevent side-effects)

- using the contraceptive pill who also take the St John's wort preparation to stop taking the St John's wort preparation as it may stop the pill from working, but to continue to take the contraceptive pill as normal

- HIV positive and on treatment and are also taking a St John's wort preparation to stop taking the St John's wort preparation and see the doctor who may suggest that the HIV viral load is checked.

Those already taking medicine who would like to start taking a St John's wort preparation should check with the pharmacist or doctor that it is safe to do so.

Stroke Association*

I joined the Stroke Association (UK) immediately after coming out of hospital. I took some comfort that my small annual financial contribution supported the work of the association, which must raise £14 million every year to fund its work. In addition, I soon had access to the publications and newsletters it produces, and feeling part of this community helped in terms of my emotional progress and rehabilitation. Wherever you live in the world, it's likely that there will be a local stroke organisation where you can find information and support.

Stroke clubs

Stroke clubs exist in towns throughout the world. They are usually run by volunteers and have a range of uses. Unless your life has been affected by stroke, it is difficult to understand how suddenly your world seems to collapse. The trauma leaves you feeling, among other things, isolated. Stroke clubs can provide an individual or family with information through formal talks and presentations, or through simply chatting over refreshments. Attending a stroke club may provide sufferers and carers with an opportunity to have a change of scenery or establish a routine. Simply meeting other stroke survivors may prove inspirational.

Swimming*

Six months after my stroke, I was ready to add this player to my programme. However, having been a strong swimmer before the stroke, my early efforts in the pool left me with very mixed emotions. I was both frustrated that I found the activity difficult, and pleased that I was able to still swim (by swim I mean that I was able to propel myself in the water to some extent). Nevertheless, as I was aware that gentle but regular aerobic exercise, such as swimming, enhances the success of rehabilitation, I stuck with it. Swimming is an especially good activity because the water reduces pressure on joints, reduces inflammation, provides support, promotes relaxation, decreases muscle guarding and spasms, and reduces pain. In addition, besides promoting cardiovascular fitness and strengthening the respiratory muscles, it can help increase flexibility.

I decided that I would try to swim every morning from Monday through to Friday. I used flotation devices and applied the FITT guidelines and principles of training sensibly. Ten months after having started swimming I was able to sign up for a charity 'Swimathon' at my local pool. While I was only able to participate in the 'fun entry' category, I was pleased to introduce an external motivational focus to the activity, in addition to my intrinsic rehabilitation focus. In some ways, psychologically at least, I was returning to my old competitive self, and even though I was preparing for the Swimathon, I visualised that I was competing in a national swimming gala event.

See also Components of fitness, FITT guidelines, Goal setting and recognising achievement, Kinesiology, Principles of training, Positive thinking and Visualisation.

'Swiss Ball' body rolling for core strength*

This is practised on a large ball (usually called a Swiss Ball or a Power Ball) and, following specific routines that imitate the logic of the neuromuscular system, body rolling is a self-care activity that helps maintain the health of the neuromuscular and skeletal systems, as well as assisting in the control and understanding of the internal sensory experience. This was of particular importance to me, having had cerebellar damage, and I was prescribed these exercises by my physiotherapist.

See also Core strength, Kinesiology, Mirror therapy and Posture.

Sympathetic nervous system (understanding)*

The sympathetic nervous system is one of the two divisions of the autonomic nervous system (the other being the parasympathetic nervous system). It consists of fibres that leave the central nervous system, pass through a chain of ganglia near the spinal cord, and are distributed to heart, lungs, intestine, blood vessels and sweat glands. In general, this system increases heart rate, dilates the pupils, constricts the peripheral blood vessels and reduces digestive secretions.

Understanding this physiological system is a cognitive player to the game and will enhance many of the other players.

See also Parasympathetic nervous system.

Tongue to the roof of the mouth*

I place the tongue on the roof of my mouth when exercising (not swimming). This may seem an odd, and indeed trivial, attention to detail. However, there are two reasons for this. First, one of the deep neck muscles attaches to the tongue, and this practice helps to stabilise the head and minimise neck discomfort, especially during core strength work. Due to the likely cause of my stroke being a vertebral artery dissection, I have to be very careful in terms of how I look after my neck. Second, in terms of traditional Chinese medicine and chikung practice, placing the tongue on the roof of the mouth is believed to connect the two main 'energy pathways' running up the axial skeleton (called the conception and governing meridians), which increases energy flow.

See also Chikung, Core strength and Traditional Chinese medicine.

Traditional Chinese medicine*

As I have said, I am very familiar with theories of traditional Chinese medicine (TCM) as a result of my 20-year involvement in the martial arts. It is claimed by some that TCM has maintained the health and sanity of the largest population of the world for the longest period of known history. In fact, the Chinese still have more traditional medical practitioners than conventional ones, and perhaps the highest worldwide life expectancy. What is often omitted by some of the more enthusiastic TCM practitioners, however, is that it has only been since the end of World War II that TCM underwent a thorough revision and evolved into a mass healthcare system. 'The traditional medley of different schools of thought and heterogeneous practices, many of which bordered on shamanism, were unified into a more coherent system, and superstitious elements were expunged' (Ellis, Wiseman and Boss 1991, p.iii). In my opinion, TCM is not necessarily more successful than the other Eastern-based approaches I have mentioned in this book, but the Chinese have used more consistent and permanent forms of writing and recording for longer when compared to other cultures. As a result, in creating the *new* Chinese medicine, the Chinese selected those theories and treatments that had been revered over centuries and were based on a coherent rationale.

In addition, there have been some translatory problems associated with the transmission of Chinese medicine to the West, and it is very likely that the Chinese presented their new medicine in the way they imagined that the West would best accept it, and labelled it 'traditional Chinese medicine'. Whatever the case, it is clear that a vital concept to appreciate for an understanding of the TCM approach is that it is our natural birthright to cope with all types of diseases if our psychological and physiological systems are working the way they should work. TCM is based on the assumption that humans are for the most part healthy by nature, and that illness is an unnatural state. According to the TCM viewpoint, there is no such thing as an incurable disease, although a patient may be incurable if his or her disease, even a simple one, has done damage beyond a certain threshold.

Chinese medical theory, as a product of traditional Chinese culture, reflects an extraordinary sensitivity towards nature, and the TCM paradigm has remained concerned with prevention as much as it has with cure, and with psychological as much as physical illnesses. Some three hundred years ago when Western medicine employed bloodletting to treat many diseases and incarcerated the psychologically ill, the Chinese had been successfully treating physical and psychological illness for over 5000 years.

Visual therapy

Approximately 20 per cent of stroke survivors have visual impairments, which are usually addressed by occupational therapists. A common problem with vision following a stroke is a visual field cut. Following a stroke an individual may experience hemianopsia, the loss of one half of a visual field. It is possible for stroke survivors who have this to be taught some compensatory techniques to help adapt. In addition, there are new therapy interventions on the horizon, including vision restoration therapy (VRT).

Visualisation*

For over 40 years, studies have shown that visualising an activity produces small but measurable reactions in the muscles involved in the imagined activity. Sports psychologists have long recognised that visualisation, when combined with physical practice, accelerates learning and enhances performance of motor skills. It is thought that during imagination of movement certain neurological events aid performance by reinforcing co-ordination patterns in the development of motor skill. Some imaging studies have now shown that the same regions of motor cortex, basal ganglia and cerebellum are activated when visualisation is used as when physical activities are actually performed.

As I had gone through my life, my natural predisposition for how I used my time had been towards participating in physical activity and sport. My life had been firmly based around my strengths and preferences. Fortunately, however, I did not feel typecast – I recognised that I needed to work out how to develop other strengths in order to set new goals. So I used visualisation to improve my moods, my concentration, my strength and my energy levels. In addition, I was dropping things and breaking plates when I tried to place them in cupboards, so I certainly needed to improve my motor skills. I had used visualisation enough through my life-long participation in sports and the martial arts, to give the concept what I thought would be a good attempt. I visualised myself as I wanted to be. I wanted to be mentally alert, emotionally calm, physically fit, physically healthy and physically strong.

Specifically, I needed to concentrate on the role of my cerebellum but I found it difficult to use other people's suggestions for guided visualisation, of which there are many available. Instead, I needed to use my own words and mental pictures. I remembered a study I had read at university which advocated the use of visualisation to help cancer patients. They were encouraged to visualise the cancer cells as weak and the white blood cells as strong. As the visualisation intensified with each session, the white blood cells were visualised as actually absorbing, or at least driving out, the cancer cells from the body. From what I could remember, this method, in combination with other medical methods of treating illness, proved successful in some cases. In my case, I created mental pictures of the result I wanted as if it had already occurred. I visualised the neurones in my brain working effectively to the point of actually re-routing messages around the area of dead brain cells. I visualised co-ordinated movement. In the beginning, I just visualised relatively straightforward daily tasks such as getting out of a chair and walking. As time went on, I visualised more complex activities, such as swimming and catching. I supported this with core strength work under the guidance of my physiotherapist and treatment from my massage therapist. I tried to fill my images with colours, sounds, smells, textures and even taste, and in so doing stimulate my senses simultaneously.

As well as visualising biomechanical aspects improving, I visualised where I wanted to be over a period of ever-increasing timescales in the future. This involved visualising as many aspects of my life as I had made decisions about. The categories seemed to choose themselves: my lifestyle, my home life, my work, my responsibilities, my finances, my diet and my 'miscellaneous' needs. I used weeks, months and years as indicators. Even though it was hard at times, I made every effort to keep the visualisation positive. Negative thoughts were of little use, and so I worked towards positive, affirmative goals. I worked towards moving nearer to what I wanted, and not just away from what I did not want. This whole process is non-competitive and becomes easier with practice. As with the breathing player, it can be performed lying, sitting, standing or moving.

Only time will tell how effective this process has been for me, but the early indications are good. In any event, the process gave me confidence and the belief that I was still, or even more, in control of me life. I tried to recognise the by-products of my daily routine. In time, I was able to affirm my ability to cope and possibly re-programme my mind back into one that was confident and vibrant.

See also Breathing, Chikung, Goal setting and recognising achievement, Kinesiology, Positive thinking, Posture, Self-hypnosis and Traditional Chinese medicine.

Walking*

Walking is an excellent activity to be employed in the prevention of stroke and, if it proves possible, is equally good as part of a rehabilitation programme. In one study (Lamontagne and Fung 2004), patients who walked at a fast speed bearing their full weight increased their gait speed by an average of 165 per cent.

I was able to walk outdoors and with attention to other players, e.g. the FITT guidelines, Posture and Principles of training benefited greatly from this player.

Yoga

Yoga originates from the Sanskrit word *yug*, which implies harnessing energies through sustained effort. Therefore, authentic yoga is a series of exercises that are intended to energise and relax the body, while also harmonising the mind, body and spirit. The use of physical postures, or *asana*, is the starting point for many people and the aspect most immediately thought of in Western societies.

In terms of stroke rehabilitation, a qualified yoga instructor will be able to introduce safe practice to stroke survivors who are confined to bed or a chair. However, it is of paramount importance that the underlying causes of the stroke are shared between doctor, patient and yoga instructor. It may be that head inversion is contraindicated, and any poses where the head drops below the waist are best avoided. In addition, the risk of vertebral arterial dissection should be considered. In this case, any spinal twist should not be taken all the way into the neck. It may be that a yoga session will predominantly focus on breathing, relaxation and visualisation players.

~ Chapter 11 ~

Financial Matters

This chapter is largely related to my experience and, therefore, that of someone living in the United Kingdom. Financial aid, homecare, disability aids and equipment, meal delivery, carers, community support networks vary from country to country, sometimes even from region to region within a country. Eligibility depends on a range of factors, including the individual's financial situation before the stroke. However, many countries have similar schemes, support networks and the opportunity to purchase private insurance policies. Generally, individual needs can be catered for and specialist advice is available.

There are two main issues associated with financial matters. In this chapter, I focus on the financial support that is available through the state and private insurance policies. The second area is concerned with the stroke survivor who may be unable to handle financial concepts in the long term and needs assistance. In such instances the law relating to the power of attorney should be considered, and it may be necessary for a friend, partner or family member to take legal advice. Whatever the case, I hope that this section will be of use and interest to all readers.

State benefits

Just knowing what is available and what an individual or family may be entitled to apply for is confusing, especially if someone is unfamiliar with the 'benefit system'. The UK has benefits that may be applicable to stroke survivors, but the onus is definitely on the individual to find out what is available. The amount of help given will very much depend on the level of need, is often means tested and may range from residential care to the cost of taking a holiday. Some financial support may be paid direct to the service provider and some may be paid directly to the stroke survivor. The benefits include the provision of equipment for the home, income support benefit, incapacity benefit, invalid care allowance, disabled person's tax credit and the disability living allowance. Similar provisions will be available in other countries. This area can get complicated, so it is best to consult with an adviser in the country of residence. To this end, I have included a variety of contact organisations and addresses at the end of this book.

Statutory sick pay (SSP)

Statutory sick pay (SSP) is a benefit which may be paid to an individual who falls ill to a physical or mental disablement. A self-employed or unemployed person cannot claim SSP. It is a benefit paid to a person in employment who is earning at least £82 a week. SSP is paid only when the individual has been sick for more than three days (usually working days). The employer is responsible for paying SSP, which can last for up to 28 weeks. There are some variables, including when the individual has reached the end of a contract of employment, goes abroad outside of the European Economic Community, is receiving statutory maternity pay or maternity allowance, is over pensionable age on the first day of sickness, has not actually started work, is affected by a strike, and is in legal custody. The National Insurance Contributions office of HM Revenue and Customs is responsible for any disputes concerning entitlement to SSP. SSP is payable at a standard rate of £68.20 per week on earnings of £82 per week or more. It is a flat rate benefit with no additions or dependants. If an individual is still ill after this time they can apply for incapacity benefit, providing they have paid enough National Insurance.

As a school teacher, I was fortunate that my employer, provided any absence was supported medically, paid me six months' full pay followed by six months' half pay. This placed me in a better position than many when I was faced with the physical and emotional trauma of stroke just before reaching the peak of my earning potential. Some individuals, especially those who are self-employed, can be faced with their income coming to an abrupt end.

Incapacity benefit

When my pay was reduced to half pay, and it was clear that I would not be returning to work in the immediate future, I received forms relating to incapacity benefit. Again, when supported with the appropriate medical reports, this offered a little extra income as Anne and I planned and coped with the reduction in monthly income.

I did receive an application pack for disability living allowance, but on seeing the amount of paperwork, I filed it away. However, if this is something that you may be eligible for, it would be worth looking into.

Private policies

Despite the very supportive and concrete financial support in terms of the SSP and incapacity benefit, I also had some private financial policies that I had been paying into for some years.

I am so very fortunate that I received, duly considered and then followed, sound financial advice several years before the stroke, while in my twenties. I still remember the conversation with my friend and independent financial consultant, Paul Fielding of Cambria Financial, about income protection policies and critical illness cover. Perhaps even more appropriately, I remember that during a financial 'sort out' the year before my stroke I nearly cancelled them all in a bid to economise! I should clarify that when I took them out, many people would have considered them a waste of money. I was in my twenties; I was at my peak of physical fitness; I had a good job with unquestionable job security; I had absolutely no health risk factors to consider; and I was 99 per cent certain that nothing would happen to me. The 1 per cent left was simply knowing that nothing in life is for certain, and thinking that it was likely that I would one day injure myself skiing, this was enough for Paul to persuade me to consider such personal insurance plans.

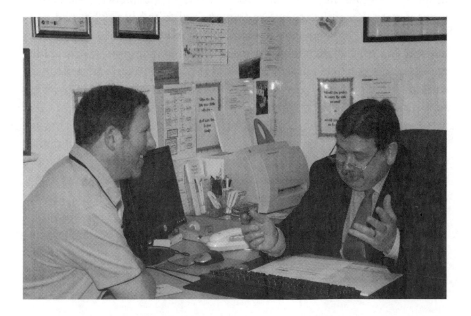

Me trying to make light of financial matters with Paul, my financial adviser

A financial payout does not make you better. However, in my case, these appropriate policies, taken out with established and reputable companies, blunted much of the financial pressure and afforded Anne and me the luxury of being able to dismiss financial worries completely during my immediate recovery from the stroke. Furthermore, I then had a little short-term financial freedom, which allowed me to reassess my earning potential and the ability to pursue a change of career. Worrying about money is the last thing a family or individual needs when a stroke or other serious life event affects the financial status quo. Some stroke survivors have had to return to work too early in terms of their recovery (however, this undoubt-edly affirms feelings of self-worth and a speedy return is the goal of many); others have had to give up their previous job; and many have had to sell their homes due to an inability to return to work and a subsequent lack of income.

Critical illness

This was the most significant of the policies I had taken out on Paul's advice. I remember him telling me that I should consider it a financial pri-ority. A supplement to my life cover, for which I paid an extra (very small) monthly premium, this gave me a tax-free one-off payment. It was several months after the stroke when I contacted Paul to tell him what had hap-pened to me. He immediately referred me back to the policy and assisted me with the paperwork and claim form. Within two months, the insurance company had contacted my doctors, received confirmation of the nature of the stroke and paid me the sum assured, which, as is typical for individuals in my position, was for the amount of my mortgage.

There is normally a one-year cut-off in terms of submitting a claim, but I am aware of at least one stroke survivor who successfully claimed on her critical illness policy more than a year after the stroke. While this payment will be made, even in the event of a good recovery, you should be aware that each insurance company will have its own payment and exclusion criteria relating to critical illness and that transient ischaemic attacks will not be covered. The small print should be checked closely as there are many exclu-sion clauses. In terms of critical illness premiums, smokers pay a hefty price for their habit. In addition, taking out a further critical illness policy when one has been redeemed becomes complex and expensive.

Income protection

My time in hospital following the major spinal surgery I had in my mid-twenties prompted me to take this policy out. I had, therefore, already taken out this policy when I met Paul for the first time. As you would expect, my policy had an exclusion clause written in that was associated with any further spinal problem I might have. Although the operation was a success, I was considered to have a pre-existing condition when I applied for the policy. However, I had insisted on a policy that would pay out if I was unable to continue with my occupation as opposed to any occupation. Paul kindly checked the policy and exclusion clause over for me and was satisfied that it was satisfactory. In my case, due to my guaranteed SSP, I had opted to accept a 52-week deferral period on any successful claim. In other words, if at any time I was still unable to return to work 52 weeks after being off work and the reason was accepted by the insurance company (an income protection policy claim must also be supported with medical evidence), it would be then that I would receive the first payment. This, I figured, would coincide with when my sick pay would cease. For this deferral period, I had paid a slightly reduced monthly premium. If the claim is successful, the policy pays a regular income for as long as the policy-holder is unable to work.

My claim was successful, and 52 weeks after the stroke this income protection policy made up most of my monthly income when my sick pay stopped completely. The amount I received each month was nowhere near what I had been receiving on half pay as it was associated with what my salary had been when I started the policy over ten years earlier. However, it had paid for itself after a mere ten weeks. I could have increased the cover in line with any pay increases, but had opted not to do so (and increase my monthly premiums at the same time) each time Paul and I reviewed it. For anyone in employment considering such a policy, it is worth checking first as some employers will have this cover with their work benefit package.

There are regular reports and letters in the financial pages of the newspapers claiming that insurers will do almost anything not to pay out. This is not my experience, and to minimise such problems you should:

- buy a policy through an independent financial adviser, who will advise on the most appropriate plan in the marketplace

- in terms of an income protection policy, read the small print relating to the occupation that cannot be done in the event of a claim

- make sure policies offer guaranteed payments or premiums

- not over-insure.

Holiday insurance

It is possible to take out travel insurance after a stroke, or with a pre-existing medical condition. Anyone taking out travel insurance should disclose any ongoing medical condition, as insurance companies are unlikely to meet claims arising from undeclared conditions. They may even reject claims for unrelated health matters if they find out about an undeclared condition. The advice is to volunteer information, even if the insurer doesn't ask for it. It may be that the first company approached will refuse cover for anyone with a pre-existing medical condition. Others may offer cover, which excludes anything relating to the pre-existing medical condition, which is not recommended. Further research will lead to companies that will offer cover, albeit at a higher premium. In such cases, opting out of baggage cover if this is covered within a home contents policy can reduce the premiums.

When a small group of family or friends are travelling together, a useful piece of advice is to insure the whole travelling party under the same policy. This will ensure that if any member of the group is taken ill and has to return to the UK, costs may be covered for the whole group.

Those travelling with someone with a pre-existing condition like stroke should also inform the insurer if it is possible that any deterioration in the individual's health may lead to a curtailing or cancelling of the holiday. Even if the stroke survivor is not going on the holiday, but a relative or carer is, many policies state exclusions relating to persons who are not travelling but on whose health the trip could depend.

In terms of medical cover, good policies should offer £1 million in Europe and £2 million in the rest of the world. They should also offer legal expenses and cover for both cancellation and curtailment of the trip.

There are some brokers who specialise in insurance for those with medical problems. In the UK, these include:

- Holiday Services
  www.askaboutinsurance.info

- Marrs Insurance Brokers
  www.marrs.co.uk

- AllClear
  www.allcleartravel.co.uk

- Free Spirit
  www.free-spirit.com

- Medicover
  www.medi-cover.co.uk

In addition, the Stroke Association Insurance Services has recently been formed and can tailor schedules to the needs of those affected by stroke. The UK number is 01603 828396.

Planning ahead

Many societies are heading towards an ageing population. People are living longer but, due to stroke and other illnesses, are not necessarily in the best of health. The result is that many people live in long-term care homes. While in some countries such as the UK the state will pay the fees for the worst off in financial terms, the majority of residents must pay the fees themselves. To do this many sell their homes or take out insurance policies to cover fees, which can average £2000 per month. Such policies cover care costs until death. The options include pre-paid policies with regular premiums, which are under review in the UK, or an immediate needs plan. The immediate needs plan can be purchased with a lump sum when required but is expensive, taking around four years to pay for itself. As with all policies, appropriate advice should be sought. In the UK, independent financial consultants and the Care Funding Bureau will offer good advice. In addition, the Stroke Association (UK) has produced a new Planning Ahead pack to help stroke patients and their families understand and cope with some of the legal procedures that can help vulnerable people exercise greater control over their finances and future. Stroke associations in other countries around the world also offer financial advice and support.

Returning to work

Due to the individual nature of stroke, some survivors within working age can return fully to work, others may return part-time, while others have to retire from their job through ill health. That is not to say that the latter will never work again, just that the type of job and the demands on the individual will be very different. The goal of returning to work may be achieved in weeks or months, or may take years. Some retraining, or a completely new career, may be required. This will be seen as a new opportunity by some, and no doubt as a lost opportunity by others. Some will be anxious about the thought of returning to work. Others will be anxious at the thought of not returning to work. The stroke survivor will be questioning their desire and ability to return to work. Again, there are a range of people and groups that are available to help and advise on such matters. These include the employer's human resources representative, possibly a worker's union, a Citizens' Advice Bureau, and a state disability employment adviser. For some, careful calculations in terms of how much can be earned and how different amounts affect benefits will be necessary, while for others, the specific skills and type of social interaction will need to be considered carefully.

In the UK, further enquiries about the Permitted Work Scheme may be appropriate to some as this may allow some work to be undertaken without the loss of any state benefits being received. Unfortunately, the rules are quite complex, with various categories of permitted work and amounts that can be earned before a loss of benefits.

For many stroke survivors, there need not be an end to having hopes and aspirations. The key is in understanding how to make adjustments to those hopes and aspirations that exist from the pre-stroke life, and how to establish new ones.

Conclusion

I hope that reading this book has proved to be an uplifting, interesting and at times educational experience. I have enjoyed writing it, as both a literary project and a means of contributing to my own recovery. Typing reasonably quickly has sometimes been difficult due to co-ordination problems, while spelling has also proved difficult at times of confusion, although some of my former teachers and recent colleagues would say that I was unable to spell correctly before my stroke! Often, I have re-read my notes finding that familiar words have been completely misused and I have found that essential words that I thought I had typed had been omitted entirely. Though short-term memory loss is common after stroke, I think that my problems were a result of the confusion and disorientation I suffered by having the stroke, and were not caused by permanent neurological changes.

It is not possible to overestimate the significance of having a stroke in the average person, whether they are a child, young adult or an elderly member of society. The medical profession often categorise strokes as being mild, moderate or severe. While I understand the medical need to categorise degrees of illness in order to establish appropriate schedules for treatment and research, it is absurd for a stroke survivor to be made to feel categorised in this way. I can assure anyone that there is nothing mild or moderate about a permanent brain injury. With this in mind, I am grateful that people like Kirk Douglas and Robert McCrum had the courage to share their experiences and emotions with me. In addition, survivors' stories such as those included in Appendix I, and such as are often posted on the websites of the Stroke Association and Different Strokes, have also been a help to me at a time of need. In a telephone conversation with a stroke survivor while researching this book, I was nervous about discussing my ideas and I described myself as 'arrogant in thinking I could write a book on such a sensitive subject'. He told me to stop thinking like that immediately, as just talking to him on the telephone lifted his spirits.

The illness of stroke, like many other serious illnesses, is a great equaliser in life. I have learnt more about myself in the months since January 2004 than I would have thought possible; and while the experience has been difficult to deal with, it has been immensely empowering. Having won my battle against a loss of confidence and succeeding in getting this book published, if people can get just one positive thing out of this book and take it with them through life, I will feel that I have made a valuable contribution to society.

As I have learnt more about the illness of stroke through the accounts of others I keep asking myself (and those closest to me ask me the same questions): Has the stroke changed me? Am I different as a result of the stroke? What about the future? I think a sensible analogy would be between my experience and that of a car journey. Pre-stroke, I was driving in my car and without realising it I was starting to hurry to complete the journey and was failing to make the most of it. I was heading towards a set of green traffic lights with the intention of going straight ahead at the junction. As the lights suddenly changed to red an emergency stop proved essential. In reality my emergency stop was the stroke. Perhaps it was my body's way of preventing something further, with more devastating consequences, as a failure to stop at the lights might have resulted in death or serious physical injury. My period of recovery has been equivalent to the time spent sitting at the junction, reflecting on the near miss, waiting for the lights to change back to green. Now that the lights have eventually changed, instead of continuing on my journey and following the same route as before, I have now decided to take a right turn and may actually end up somewhere else. By making the turn I am now on a slower route. I now pass more people. I now have more experiences and am actually still travelling. Unlike the car journey, while I am not sure I have any real control over the length of my life, I certainly feel that I have been empowered to be brave enough to change direction, to travel at my own pace and make myself (and anyone who may now be in the car with me) as important as the journey itself.

With this in mind, my motives for writing this book have not included a desire for pity or profit. I have written this book merely because I have found that I can. This in itself is something I am very grateful for. I have been given an opportunity to reflect, something the pace of 21st-century life does not readily allow. I hope that some of you will be encouraged to do the same. Slow down before the body decides to make an emergency stop. To revert to the analogy, there are those who will already have overshot the lights and may be recovering from a collision at the junction. In the hope that I do not sound patronising or condescending, I would say that it's never too late to continue on the journey, even if it is by foot and the path doesn't lead you to the destination you originally intended. Take everything in, stop and talk, arrange to meet friends and loved ones on the way and only look back to remind you of the route that lies ahead.

From reading about strokes in the months that followed mine, I realise that I am indeed very lucky. I received early medical attention as the result of action by my friends. I received an early brain scan and I was stable and under constant nursing care for the first seven days. I have also learnt that while the human brain is not giving up its secrets easily and is so complex that it may never be successful in comprehending itself, fortunately the medical profession is still learning about it. As a result, the illness of stroke is now regarded more and more as the emergency that it is. This is something that was not happening as recently as 20 years ago when, by and large, stroke patient assessment and care was nihilistic as it was thought that very little could be done. The personal, social and political implications of this should not be underestimated. Educating the public to treat stroke as a 'brain attack' and to seek emergency treatment is a crucial and urgent requirement for society. For every minute lost, from the onset of symptoms to the time of emergency contact, the limited window of opportunity for intervention is reduced. The longer the delay in seeking medical attention, the more damage a stroke can do, and the less recovery can be achieved. Robert McCrum lay alone at home for many hours before he managed to alert people to his situation.

That said, scientists, researchers and the medical profession are gaining an ever-increasing understanding of both the workings of the brain and the relationship between brain and mind. However, even with medical advances the general public still need to be reminded of the simple things relating to the illness of stroke. Increasing society's and individuals' under-standing of the warning signs of a stroke and how to respond can mean the difference between death and survival for some who fall victim to the illness.

As I have said, I am lucky to have made a significant recovery from a cerebellar stroke, which can prove fatal. I am lucky that the emergency services were able to respond relatively promptly and that I was given oxygen so quickly. I am lucky that the A&E doctor was not too proud to ask for a second opinion, which resulted in my admission to hospital. I am lucky that I had the CT scan on my first day in hospital so my case was clear from the start (a Royal College of Physicians' audit of stroke care in 2004 found that 53 per cent of suspected UK stroke victims wait over 48 hours for a scan). I am lucky to have had the love and care of my parents, and of Anne and her family. I am lucky to have the support of my friends and the understanding of my former colleagues. In the same way that the onset of stroke varies, so does the aftermath. This leaves some, like me, with virtually a complete recovery of sensation and movement, and others with permanent and severe disability. That said, most stroke victims seem to recover to a state somewhere between the two extremes.

Our mind, body and spirit all meet in our beliefs and actions. What I believe has greatly affected how I have approached my recovery. I believe that my recovery has been a consequence of my outlook. As we get older, we become more self-assured, so events like strokes can have even greater impact on our self-confidence. However, it seems to me that our individual sense of identity is resilient and, that when challenged, it can be built on and developed. I have always felt that fate acted around me, and that every-thing happens, at a specific time, for a definite purpose. The real challenge is in interpreting accurately what this purpose is, and in establishing goals and accepting that it will be impossible to determine whether or not the interpretation is correct. I have therefore changed my mind to some extent, and now think that I have more of a direct hand in what happens and am more of an influence than fate.

In my case, rather then be filled with regret about having had a sudden stroke at a young age, I now actually spend more time concerned about what opportunities I would have wasted, and experiences I would not have ahead of me, if I had not experienced it. Simply speaking, as I strove to get better, I sought both independence and interdependence. As I have applied the various players to my daily life, I have no doubt that, somehow, and in many ways, my life will be better for having experienced the stroke. I appreciate what I have a whole lot more, and I have reaffirmed some good qualities – so far, I am still not a quitter. Like most people, when things do not go to plan, I hear a little voice inside my head telling me 'You're nothing special. Why should things get better for you? Why challenge yourself so much when you are likely to fail?' When I hear it, I remind myself that I would show commitment to and support my friends and family if they needed it, and therefore I really should show the same commitment to myself.

So, in addition to working on this book, I took a course and passed my advanced driving test with the Institute of Advanced Motorists; trained as a clinical hypnotherapist with the BST Foundation; qualified as a licensed neurolinguistic programming (NLP) practitioner under NLP co-founder Dr Richard Bandler; attended a short business course; started my own busi-ness; and introduced the added complication of actually trying to write two books at the same time. Embarrassed about telling anyone I was trying to write this book, and in order to justify to Anne the time spent at the desk, I have also worked on a book for martial art practitioners. This was an interesting development in terms of my recovery. I started to write the second book, not as someone recovering from a stroke, but as a completely fit, 'unaffected', athlete and researcher. On reflection, I am convinced that the fact I was not totally psychologically immersed in being a recovering stroke survivor actually helped drive me to take as much responsibility for my own recovery as possible. I made an effort to write in a disciplined way, and in so doing continued to use left-brain activity. This may have had the effect of inhibiting slightly the more negative emotional responses associated with largely right-brain activity. At the time of writing this I am pleased to say that there is some interest in my other work, and it too may one day be published.

Suffering a stroke (or other major life event) strips a person bare and leaves them vulnerable. It can take a person close to actually losing the essence of who they are. However, surviving a stroke (or other major life event) can actually strengthen the essence of who they are. Similarly, the process of rebuilding, which is undeniably challenging, can be stimulating, informative and empowering. I have now come through the bewilderment that the stroke left me with, and having survived it I know that the experience has empowered me to make brave decisions rather than just talk about them as I may have done before the stroke. I have devoted some of my recovery time to creating opportunities for myself. I decided during my time at home not to abdicate responsibility for my health or quality of life. While aspects of 21st-century living and society can sometimes seem to have a natural inclination towards chaos, ill health and decay, I still have a free will and, importantly, potential. I have consciously set myself objectives outside of the limits I thought possible. This culminated in the setting up of my business, AMCAN Consultancy & Training Ltd. Anne suggested the name, because as well as being a shortened version of my name, *amcan* is the Welsh word for 'goal' or 'purpose'. I hope to use my skills (both old and new) and reflect on my life experiences to help others identify their own sense of purpose and achieve their own goals. I renew my commitment to striving for a better life, every day, and there are no short cuts to doing this. You either choose to do it, or you don't. It really is a simple choice.

I now appreciate the health I have, the opportunities I still have before me, my relationships with my family, Anne and my friends, and the simpler, important things that define me as an individual. I now understand myself a whole lot better and believe that a new chapter is just beginning…

Survivors' Stories

The following words are unedited. They are the words used by stroke survivors, who have kindly let me include them in this book. They are inspirational real stories and describe real feelings. They illustrate many of the points raised in this book and, the order in which I have included them, reflect the various aspects of stroke as they appear in this book.

Shakila Khan, 18

I had my stroke at the age of 18. A large area of my left cerebral was damaged from an arterial bleed that left the right side of my body completely paralysed with total loss of speech.

This incident happened at around 9am one May morning, while I was standing on a bus for my daily work at the University College Hospital Pharmacy Department, where I was a trainee Pharmacy Technician. I had a severe headache, but my thoughts at the time were about oncoming A Level exams in a few weeks' time. Then I heard the conductor saying, 'Fares, please.' I held out my hand with my money but I could not talk. Then I felt a cold sensation in my head, I touched my face and head to feel if they were wet but they were dry. My eyes could not focus anymore. I was holding the passenger handle tightly as I felt a loss of balance at the same time. I wanted to scream but the sound just would not come out.

I heard a voice saying, 'Sit down', apparently to me but my eyes were going to close and I could not see where to sit. My body was out of control and I was frightened and confused about what was happening to me. Then I vomited all over myself. I heard an ambulance siren and after that I became unconscious.

My family had been looking for me everywhere for three days until they were told by the police that I was at the Prince of Wales Hospital. Since I was unconscious, the doctors assumed that I was on drugs (instead of thinking of other possible reasons) and they waited for me to regain consciousness. Both the doctors and nurses told my family that I was going to recover even after they were told by my family that I never took drugs.

It was on my family's third visit to the hospital and after seeing no improvement in my condition that my sister tried to stimulate my body for any response. She felt that the right side of my body was very cold and heavy compared to the left side. She thought it rather unusual and she went to tell the doctor. The doctor-in-charge immediately came to check for body responses. She suspected something and called the consultant very urgently. On spotting the symptom, they quickly made arrangements for an immediate transfer to The National Hospital for Nervous Diseases.

As soon as I arrived at the hospital I was taken to have a brain scan. Then the doctors broke the bad news to my family – that I had less than 30 per cent chance of recovery because the blood clot had damaged a large area of my brain cells due to the delay in diagnosis. This was another blow to my family as they had not imagined that it could get any worse. The doctors told them that they were unable to operate and stop the bleeding while I was still unconscious.

In the next few days, I regained consciousness and was operated on. After the operation and the intensive care, general care and then the initial rehabilitation programme started. Six months later I was transferred to the Homerton Hospital in Hackney, where I began to feel conscious of my disability for the first time. I felt miserable, angry, frustrated and on top of that, the staff did very little to encourage me to get better.

I was transferred to an outpatient Rehabilitation Centre after about four months, where the staff were encouraging and helpful. The speech, occupational and physiotherapist in the centre stirred me towards the independence that I enjoy now! I passed my driving test and now I can go everywhere without help. I also went to the local college to learn computer literacy, photography, drama and how to make videos. Now, I am doing photography and performing arts. Some of my friends have asked why I don't go back to my old job as a Pharmacy Technician. I say to them that I want to forget about the past and want to start a new life, and besides there are many other areas to explore! I have made new friends, found new interests and hobbies. I have done voluntary work with Cancer Research and Different Strokes briefly, which I found a very rewarding experience. I have been to Kashmir twice on holiday and found it very peaceful and close to nature. I travelled to America and Canada last winter. Then in the summer I went to North Wales to make an attempt to climb Snowdonia! Now, I take each day as it comes. I do not make too many plans. I have become much closer to God after this experience than ever before and I definitely believe in destiny.

Nicola Sawyer-Roskell, 24

I've come to realise in the past four years that you should never take life for granted. I thought I was a very healthy person. I had a great job as a neonatal nurse, a great fiancé, a lovely home and I had no clue that anything about my life would ever change unexpectedly.

In 2000 I started a new job in Leicester. I was really enjoying it, the ward was nice, my colleagues were lovely and the job was what I'd always wanted to do. An added perk was that my manager had paid for me to do a neonatal management course, starting in May, which would lead to promotion. My fiancé and I were planning our dream wedding for June and looking forward to our honeymoon in Bali. To help pay for it I was working plenty of shifts as we'd just bought our first home together too so you could say I was a little bit busy! Every day off I was either travelling to Yorkshire to organise the wedding or studying. I was having a lot of bad migraines, due to the tiredness and the stress, which left me almost blind. I wasn't looking after myself very well and I lost weight and got a few spots. I was horrified! We'd paid a fortune for our wedding photographer and I wasn't going to be a spotty bride!

I went to see my doctor and he told me I should try taking a form of the pill (Dianette). I refused as my school friend had died from a stroke whilst taking the pill. He reassured me and packed me off with my little bag of pills without asking my medical history or taking my blood pressure.

Two weeks later (with lovely clear skin!) my fiancé, Tom, smuggled me along on a business trip to Liverpool as I needed a couple of days off. I felt quite odd – weepy and depressed and not my usual self. When Tom finished work we went to the hotel bar. I began to feel quite ill, really exhausted, sick, and thirsty but somehow couldn't drink. I went to bed early and thought I'd sleep it off but the next day I still wasn't right. We went home and I had another early night as my mum, sister and sister-in-law-to-be were coming over for a bridesmaid dress fitting the next day and I wanted to shake off whatever I was coming down with.

At around 3am I started having a very weird dream. I wasn't sure if it was real or not. I woke up to find I had a headache and pins and needles in my fingers and toes and the right side of my face was numb. I thought I'd been lying funny and lay there trying to get the blood flowing again. I had what I thought was a terrible migraine as well, I couldn't see. It was as if someone had shone a bright light into my eyes and blinded me. I decided I'd go downstairs and get my migraine tablets once the strange feeling had worn off but it seemed to be getting worse and spreading up my legs and along my arm and the feeling was going altogether in my hands and feet. Stupidly I didn't want to wake Tom up in case I worried him so I lay there panicking quietly and feeling like my head would explode with my body becoming more and more numb. I began to think maybe this was a bit more than a migraine as I was feeling very 'distant' and not sure what was real and not. I thought I was going to black out and my crying woke Tom up. When he asked what was wrong I tried to tell him but it was as if I'd had an anaesthetic at the dentist's. One side of my mouth was not moving and my speech was slurred. I blurted out something about not having any feeling and amazingly Tom understood and scooped me up and carried me downstairs to phone an ambulance. He called NHS Direct first as I'd told him there was probably nothing wrong really and I didn't want to go to hospital in case people from work saw me! The woman on the end of the phone said 'I'm sending an ambulance – this sounds like she's had a stroke.' I told Tom she must have written my date of birth down wrong. I was 24, stupid woman! Only old people have strokes. Phone her back, tell her! He said it'd be better if I did get checked over so I reluctantly agreed on condition he helped me get dressed because I wasn't going in in my dressing gown!

I got into the ambulance alone and left Tom to get my things. I began to cry again and the paramedic reassured me that I'd be fine and that she'd seen a girl just like me a couple of weeks ago and she had had a hemiplegic migraine. She'd had a sleep and woken up fine the next morning. 'Thank God!' I thought. 'That's what I've got and I'm going to be fine!'

The doctors in A&E were in no rush to see me. They arranged a CT scan, which I was told was fine. No one seemed to know what to do with me. The staff seemed convinced I'd taken something I wasn't telling them about and took blood from me after asking several times if I was really sure I hadn't taken anything. I told them my head felt like it was splitting open so they gave me a couple of Paracetamol. I felt they hadn't really understood what I was telling them! In the end they agreed with the paramedic, it was a hemiplegic migraine, and after a few hours' observation on a ward sent me home as I could now manage a few wobbly steps alone, although I couldn't feel my leg, and my arm was like I was carrying someone else's arm about attached to my body. I was really relieved to be leaving as my visitors had now turned up and I didn't want to be stuck in hospital when there were wedding things to sort out.

My mum came to visit me on the ward and pestered the doctors about doing more tests. I told her to leave them alone as I was desperate to get home to my own bed where I'd feel much better after a night's sleep and everything would be okay. My mum called a taxi for us and packed my bags. Tom had gone back to work after being reassured I was fine. I began to feel really unwell. The room was spinning and I felt very confused and like I was going to black out but still I wanted to go home and in my strange state of mind that was more important than letting someone know how ill I felt, besides, this was just a migraine and I didn't want to look stupid by making a fuss.

I got in the Taxi and gave him directions to my old house I'd lived at 8 months ago, luckily my mum knew where I lived and put him right. Waves of lightheadedness and nausea were coming over me and I had to fight hard to stay conscious. The driver was trying to chat to me but my answers didn't make much sense. I was trying to act normal so I didn't scare my mum but it was probably too late for that. I got home and dragged myself up the stairs with one arm. I had never felt so tired or ill in all my life and I had to go and have a sleep. I was asleep as soon as my head hit the pillow – it was around 4pm and I didn't come round until 7am ish when Tom got up for work. He asked if I was okay and I gave my usual mumbled response so off he went. After a further 3 hours of sleep with more strange dreams and not being sure if I was awake or not I decided to get up and see if I was 'working' again. I slid out of bed and collapsed in a heap onto the floor. My visitors were in the lounge below and my mum came to see if I was alright. I had now completely lost the feeling all down my right side and couldn't move it at all. The paramedics were back again, carrying me down the dog-leg staircase on a stretcher seemed hilariously funny to me although probably not to them! I was still very confused and thought I was in the ambulance alone although my sister insists she was with me all the way. I cried my eyes out once I was in the ambulance – I couldn't seem to control my emotions at all.

The doctors repeated the tests – all normal for someone having a paraplegic migraine apparently. They sent me off to a general medical ward in time for lunch. It was parked in front of me with a knife and fork and I was left to it. I couldn't cut the food, take the lid off my drink, or reach the buzzer which had been put to my right, so I sat and cried like a baby until they came to take my tray away, whilst the elderly ladies in the rest of the beds pretended not to notice. I told the nurse I couldn't eat as I needed it to be cut for me at which she rolled her eyes and said 'Can't you cut it yourself?' She reluctantly did it for me once I explained what was wrong but I couldn't eat anyway. I couldn't tell whether I was chewing food or my mouth and I kept choking. That was probably the first time I thought about the possibility of me being like this permanently and I was petrified. I had clung onto the thought I'd wake up and be back to normal and it didn't seem likely somehow when I was getting so much worse. To me it seemed like I'd had a stroke but I told myself I didn't have any risk factors – I was too young, too healthy, didn't drink (not much anyway!) and didn't smoke, hadn't ever taken drugs and wasn't over-weight, but the thought of my friend and the pill at the back of mind was ringing alarm bells.

I was put on the ward on Good Friday so there weren't any specialists on duty or physios and I was pretty much left to my own devices. No more tests, just the usual blood pressure tests every few hours. There wasn't even a TV on the ward to stop the boredom and with only one arm to work the wheelchair I'd been put in I tended to get a bit dizzy trying to go anywhere! Almost a week later a specialist stroke nurse came to see me and checked me over. 'I'm afraid it looks like a stroke,' she told me. I don't remember her saying anything else to me as my mind was rac-ing, mostly with denial and the hemiplegic migraine diagnosis and the fact I hated her for trying to take my hope away from me.

In all the time I was in hospital no-one had tried to get me into a standing position and I'd had no physio and my right hand and foot were swelling up like balloons. I thought one of the auxillary nurses, Donna, had gone mad when she came to see me one day and said 'We're going for a walk.' I waited for the punchline but there wasn't one and she hauled me up into a standing position from the wheelchair. I was very wobbly and felt weak from being immobile for so long and it hurt to put weight on my right foot as the lightest touch sent pins and nee-dles shooting through my foot and ankle. She supported my right side and helped me to take my first few wobbly steps. I couldn't believe it! I was so happy I was in tears and hugging Donna. She became my very favourite nurse, my heroine! She came to see me and get me up and about every day and gradually I managed to get to the toilet myself, which doesn't sound like a lot, but to me, being able to use the toilet in peace was wonderful! Donna did all the girly things for me like tying my hair back for me that the other nurses seemed too busy to do but made such a huge difference to me. I felt human again after she'd tidied me up and not like the woman dribbling away in a wheelchair.

Every day Tom and my parents came in to visit me and wheeled me outside so I could hobble around the hospital grounds in the sunshine. I can never thank them enough for these visits, they're all that kept me sane and stopped me feeling so depressed.

On the return from one of my 'wanders' Donna came to see me to let me know a stroke specialist consultant was coming to see me, my Mum waited with me as Tom was still at work. He came in, did a few tests and simply said 'You've had a stroke'. He couldn't tell me if I would ever improve or give me any hope of being any better than I was. I asked if I'd see him again and he told me he was a very busy man and off he went leaving me hysterical and my mum in tears. The only thing that made me smile was the fact my mum was swearing like a trooper about him and I'd never heard her swear before! In the middle of all these tears poor Tom came in to visit and was greeted by two hysterical women who couldn't talk to tell him what was wrong. We were taken to a side room where Tom calmed me down and got some sense out of me. He was shell shocked and had lots of questions to ask but the 'very busy' consultant had gone.

Tom took me to a nearby park for a walk. I was still in tears and people must have wondered what was going on. 'I'm going to be hard work, you know. I'll understand if you don't want to marry me now.' He just laughed and called me a silly mare and reassured me that he still loved me just as much which was such a relief!

Two days later I was discharged with some aspirin to take once a day. I'd had no home assessment so it was a bit of a shock to be out of the 'cocoon' of the hospital and into the real world where stairs were now very difficult and had to be crawled up with one arm and slid down. I could no longer drive, prepare food, take a phone message or even fasten my own bra! I was pretty depressed for a while when I first got home but I had a wedding to organise and managed to keep myself busy with that.

A week after my discharge I had an MRI scan which confirmed what I already knew. It had been an ischaemic stroke in the base of my left hand side of my brain where all the signals from the left side of the brain travel into my spinal cord and to the right of my body. The pictures were amazing to look at. I seemed to be missing a fairly large chunk of grey matter in and around my hypothalamus so I feel lucky to be as well as I am.

My one hour a week with the hospital physio wasn't getting me anywhere so I booked sessions with a private physio who specialised in treating young stroke victims. After a few weeks I could walk without a limp, a few more weeks and I could move my hand and shortly after that I could write my name with my right hand. I was almost bankrupt but it was worth it! Tom and I had a wonderful wedding day and a fantastic honeymoon. I swam every day and gradually my strength started to come back. We went parasailing, which isn't something I'd have done before the stroke, and we trekked through rainforests and because I wasn't having to eat hospital food or trying to prepare my own meals, some of the weight went back on.

Thanks to Tom, my family, Donna, Jon the physio, and the birth of my miniature physio, Adam, in 2002, I'm now 90 per cent back to normal. Adam has been wonderful physio, forcing me to use my right hand by constantly finding new and exciting ways of putting himself in danger. The best medicine I've had is the laughter he creates.

I'll never go back to nursing now because I don't have the fine movement that's needed and I get tired too easily. I've moved house because of the bad memories I had in the old one and have great new friends and I'm closer to my family. I had an automatic car converted with a left foot accelerator so I'm mobile again and life is really good. I'm going to try my hand at teaching or freelance editing when I get some time to myself again but I'm going to stick to doing one thing at once this time! Tom has booked me some gliding lessons for later this year and I'm doing far more dangerous things than I would have done had I not had the stroke. Every year I have an STS day (Sod the Stroke) on its anniversary where I try to do something a bit mad (like gliding!). It's taught me life is too short to avoid doing things you're afraid of. My advice to anyone who's had a stroke is – Don't ever give up!

Harvey Brooker, 31

Mine is the malformed lump of veins and arteries (the size of a small lemon) version. All started on my mountain bike. Decided to get some fresh air to clear my head. There was this really weird sensation as though my head was expanding underneath my helmet. This was followed by a pounding headache which lying on the floor with cushions on my head didn't help.

Five days later I'm at work on the phone. Suddenly feeling very peculiar I try to call out to my boss but my mouth isn't working. Her bosom provided a comfy landing. The rest is fuzzy. An extended ambulance journey (driver confused Bradford with Bedford) and some days later I arrive at the Stroke Unit in Northampton Hospital.

Memories of falling out of bed and off toilets, accidentally throwing full bottles of urine onto my neighbour's bed (though empty) and mostly of really caring staff. Went from total left side paralysis (couldn't even wink) to kind of walking, thanks to my physio John. Arrived home thinking this is the best place in the world and remembering those unforgettable words 'upper limbs are very unreliable'.

I had plenty of time in bed to contemplate 'life'. Hadn't planned this to happen at 31 years old. In between 'enjoying' hospital cuisine and chatting with staff and 'fellow inmates' I began contemplating what all this meant. My father was a workaholic who dreamed of the day he would be made redundant. Then he could start enjoying life. He was, but didn't get a chance to. My Dad died shortly after being made redundant from motor neurone disease. This dramatically affected my outlook on life and career direction. In my mid twenties, I left selling to train to be a careers adviser. My mission to help people find work they will enjoy.

In my work with clients I have always focused on people working out what their 'values' are, the things that really matter. When lying in my bed following my stroke the thing that brought tears to my eyes most often was the thought of not being able to cuddle my wife and little girl (now 3). I had just stared a job that meant spending even more time away from home. The stroke has been a blessing in disguise. It has made me realise that it's not enough to know and talk about what is most important to you. You have got to spend your time doing it because you don't know how long you've got.

I don't play the lottery anymore because I realise I have everything I could possibly need. I now work part time and run my own small business helping people find that balance in their lives. I've gained a strong faith as a result of what has happened. On several occasions I have 'sensed' that I'm being looked after. I've also come to realise what a wonderful group of people I am surrounded by and how they matter more than anything else.

Talking of wonderful people, Amanda who has appeared in the Different Strokes magazine gave me a lot of inspiration at a time when I needed it. She came to one of the early meetings of my local group. I felt young there and gravitated toward her as she looked nearer my age. As it turned out we were the same age. She had suffered a stroke at 26 years old and was now 32. 'If she can recover that much then there's hope,' I thought.

In the same edition of the magazine there was a man who had run a marathon. Something else I was told I wouldn't do again. I've made a deal with my physio that we are going to do a 10km race together. It won't be this year but it will happen.

That's why I reckon I've had a 'stroke of luck'.

Joanne Brown, 34

My name is Joanne Brown, I am 34 years old, live in Leominster with my Partner Sean, boxer dog called George and my daughter Charlotte who is 5 years old. I work as a Telesales Operator in town selling Mail-Order Sportswear. I was taking Oral Contraception and I was a smoker.

This is my story regarding the Stroke I suffered on the 27th October 2003.

Monday 27th October 2003. I got up with Charlotte and came downstairs to make breakfast, had a coffee, put some washing on the line, had a fag, went and got dressed and I felt fine. It was half term week and my mum was going to look after Charlotte for me, as I was going to work between 12–3pm. I started the housework upstairs and my ears popped, I could not hear anything and my head felt all muzzy. I still continued to do the hoovering, thinking my ears would pop and I would be able to hear once again. When I got downstairs I started the hallway, the kitchen and finally the living room, where I found Charlotte lying on the floor colouring. I began to ask her to move her things so that I could hoover around her, but my words came out all muddled up and she could not understand me. I kept thinking what is the matter with me!!! I obviously did not know that this was a warning of what was about to happen. After a couple of seconds my speech was back to normal, and I did not think about it again.

Charlotte and I drove to my Mum's at Richards Castle, 7 miles outside of Leominster. When we got there, I was telling Mum all about what had happened that morning, and she said it sounded like the first signs of a Stroke, I said don't be so silly, I'm not old enough to have one of those as I only associated Stroke with elderly people. My Mum's neighbour and Sean's Nan had recently suffered a Stroke and they were in their eighties. I began to start sentences about other things that Charlotte and I were going to do over the half term, but could not remember the words to finish what I was saying. This was very disturbing and Mum had noticed that I was getting very annoyed with myself and told me to go and sit down in the living room. She made me another cup of coffee, which I started to drink and soon started to choke on it, as I could not swallow properly. My Dad was upstairs sleeping as he works nights, my mum went upstairs to wake him up, but he was already up, as he heard all of the commotion going on downstairs. It only felt like a couple of minutes had passed, but I could not talk at all. I still had movement in my arm and still could walk.

At that stage my Dad phoned my place of work to say that I was not going in today and also phoned the Doctors in Leominster for an appointment. We went straight to the Doctors and my sister looked after Charlotte, as she lives opposite my mum, and it was her day off. My mum was trying desperately to get hold of Sean on his mobile phone to let him know what was going on. On the way to the Doctors, my right side of my mouth was slightly drooped and all I could think about was 'what is the matter with me?' When we finally got to the doctors, my dad needed to come into the room with me as I still could not talk, as he needed to tell the Doctors about my symptoms. After a pulling and pushing exercise on my right-hand side of my body, she told me to go straight to the Hereford Hospital.

Sean took me to the hospital and when we got there, I needed to be pushed in by wheelchair as I could not walk, we went straight in to the A&E Department. Later in the afternoon my speech came back a little and the feeling in my right leg came back. Sean and I thought that I would be able to go home – how wrong we both were!!! The Doctor who was looking after me and doing lots of tests and taking lots of blood, was waiting for a bed to become available in Admissions. I was attached to a drip as I still could not swallow properly and taken up to the Admission Ward.

The next morning I was paralysed down my right-hand side of my body and could not speak at all. The Doctors came around later on that morning and told me that the symptoms I had been experiencing were a Stroke. They said I had suffered two minor TIAs on Monday morning/afternoon and a major CVA on Monday night. All I could think about was WHY ME!!! After the initial period of emotion I decided that this has happened for a reason, and I am determined to lead a normal life.

I spent a total of 4 weeks in hospital and came out on the 27th November 2003, after having loads of Speech Therapy, Physiotherapy and Occupational Therapy.

It is nearly 10 months ago since I had my Stroke. I can now talk, walk, move my right arm and do normal everyday things. I still get tired and need a nap in the afternoon, but I think I can live with that as it could have been a lot worse. The reason for my stroke was apparently a blood clot travelling up my body and finally placing itself on my left-hand side of my brain, causing the loss of speech and loss of movement in my right arm and leg. The Doctors do not know why it happened, or where the blood clot came from, and I suppose I will never know. I am thankful that I have recovered so well and pray to the gods that I don't have another one. The medication I am taking now and for the foreseeable future is 75mg of Aspirin.

If any other Stroke Survivors read my story, I hope it gives them inspiration as there is life after stroke.

Bob Smith, 42

Twelve years ago in December of 1990, I was the victim of what was termed a 'stroke'. Later diagnosis indicated that I had suffered a massive 'brainstem' stroke. This happens when communication between the brain and body has been interrupted, most likely by an aneurism or blockage in an artery. In literature from the Stroke Network site on the Internet, it is listed as 'a condition resulting from interruption of motor pathways in the ventral pons, usually by infarction'. Fancy words for saying that someone has suffered a stroke and the brain and body are not in-sync with each other. My stroke was brought about by a rupture or weakness in a blood vessel that caused blood to spill out in the area of my brainstem and caused cellular damage. Following my stroke, I had several CAT-scans and MRI's, but nothing showed up on these fancy x-rays until about four months after the actual event or accident.

Let me take you through some of the events of that night. I had no prior warnings except some dizziness and nausea for which my doctor treated as a sinus infect. There were no warnings of the impending danger. Near eleven o'clock I did feel a cold shiver run throughout my body. It started at the tip of my head and traveled all the way to the tip of my toes. It was like an electrical shock. I retired early because of extreme fatigue. I was a teacher at a college and we had just started a new semester, so I figured that was the mitigating factor in my being tired. About three o'clock in the morning, I awoke very nauseated. I went to the restroom, but really got no relief. I leaned to tell my wife of my feelings, but could only stammer to say, 'I can't move.' At that point, I collapsed onto the floor. Little did I know the severity of what was happening in my skull.

I can remember lying on the floor and being able to see everything that was going on. Why were my wife and children acting so upset? And why were these strangers in my house shining lights in my eyes and sticking stuff in me? Also, why the devil could I see, but not move or talk? The answer to these questions would be answered, but not before I spent about two and a half months in a coma. I should, by all accounts, never woken up, but I am stubborn, so I faced whatever it was that had knocked me down so hard and left me functioning only partially.

Here are some of the facts that I have learned. The spinal cord of course runs up and down the back, or spine. In a little area at the base of the brain, there are many little nerves and fibers that attach to the spinal cord and anchor it a place in brain called the cerebellum. The cerebellum is also connected to nerves that are connected with facial expressions. That is why stroke can cause a person to droop on one side of the face after a stroke. Also the cerebellum is associated with movements that utilize hand-to-eye coordination, plus controls much of the movement and balance related activities. This is the reason for such un-coordinated movement following a stroke. As I retained a sense of consciousness for a while, I could see, but was totally unable to move or respond to anyone or anything. This is referred to as 'locked-in syndrome'. Many stroke victims are wrongly diagnosed because of this high state of confusion and inability to respond orally. Because of my brainstem stroke, I had become completely paralyzed. Communication between my cerebellum and body had been interrupted, so I was subject to whatever ravages this stroke was causing.

Following the drugs and natural fogginess of a coma, I awoke to a state that was very foreign to me. I have always been the 'A' type person, always on the go, boundless energy and all. But now, I lay in bed and waited for someone to lift me. I had a tough time dealing with the aftermath of a stroke. There were times I felt very angry with everyone and everything. Other times, I was swallowed up in a pool of self-pity. Why me? I had to grieve the loss of body parts that used to respond well. Now, some of my appendages just hang lifeless and uncontrollable.

This was very hard for me to understand, because I was a gifted athlete. Coordination was my middle name, but now, tying my shoes was an impossible feat. Everything I knew had to be remapped to fit into my one-arm and hand world. Simple little feats became hard and arduous. Feelings of useless crept into every cell of my being. It became very apparent to me that my life was forever changed. All of this had happened and I did not have control.

My experiences in a rehabilitation center at Pitt Memorial Hospital in Greenville, North Carolina are varied, exciting, and disappointing to say the least. Varied, because they have taught me so many, many things necessary to survive in society. Exciting, because I have faced so many new situations and met such wonderful people. Disappointing, because I cannot do some of the things that they have shown me. Disappointing, because of the lack of ability to regain some of the paralyzed features they have so vigorously worked with me on.

There have been years of therapy, doctors' care, and study of similar brain accidents. The more I learn, the luckier I feel. People do not usually survive a severe brainstem stroke. I did survive, 'duh', being able to write this is my proof. My left side is pretty useless, but I do have some shoulder movement, and limited arm movement. My voice is now very different and monotone, but at least I communicate. I can walk fine now, but I do have a pronounced limp on my left side. Also, rest has become very necessary during any physical exertion. I am typing this now with one finger pecking, so I might make some flubs. I am able to drive my car now and I like to get out and explore. That is one thing that helps me deal with day-to-day problems. My computer has become a very dear friend. Through use and manipulation of software, I can design houses, buildings, and other projects. I can stay informed by reading a great deal of information on the Internet. I can stay in touch with family and friends electronically with email. When designing a house or something, I can be very competitive because of my computer. It does not care about my disabilities just as long as I keep pressing the right keys. My computer has become my left arm.

People can be wonderful and supportive following a stroke. Perhaps the fact that I have slowed my actions a great deal, I now have the time to realize their good intentions and motifs. I have been through an emotional roller coaster, but have withstood it all and made some really good friends. I still have a great deal of drive and determination, and that has helped me return to the point in my life of pseudo-independence and happiness. I used the term 'pseudo-independence' because I will always need people and their help. I do not proclaim that I am happy because of stroke, however, I do proclaim that I have become a much better person. It all seems a blur, but much like some one picked me out of a crowd of humanity and said 'tag – you're it'. Sure, it is terribly unfair! Others have faced such adversity and emerged from the far side better off. The National Stroke Association refers to stroke as a 'brain attack'. Surely that is a gross understatement. A stroke attacks you like nothing else. If you are lucky as I have been, you can survive and live an almost normal life. One tends to concentrate upon those activities that fit into a range of 'do-able' and stay away from those that will certainly lead to frustration and high physical demand. Please learn the warning signs of a stroke, and tell your family members and friends about the signs. You, be sure to remove any dangerous health anomalies that might tend to enhance stroke risk.

So 'tag – now you're it!'

Johnny Watts, 43

February 12th 2002: I went to bed at midnight, a very fit, healthy, non-smoking, non-drinking 43-year-old male, employed as an HGV tanker driver in the UK Petroleum Industry – 4 hours later my life had changed forever, I woke up having a serious brain haemorrhage, later to be diagnosed as an Arteriovenous Malformation (AVM). I was completely paralysed down the left side of my body – I was rushed to Hurstwood Park Neurological Hospital at Haywards Heath, where doctors told me that I was very lucky to be alive, but unfortunately there was a possibility that I may never walk, or use my arm again – LUCKY??? how could that be lucky? – that was when I decided that I wasn't going to let this illness beat me. There was a very high possibility that I would require brain surgery to remove the AVM, but this could not be accessed until the blood clot had dispersed naturally, so after 4 weeks at Hurstwood Park, I was transferred to Southlands Rehab Hospital at Shoreham – during the next 12 weeks I was allowed to start a 'light' rehabilitation programme, and underwent numerous tests including Angiograms, CT scans and MRI scans, all confirming that embolisation treatment would not be possible, and that I would need a Craniotomy (brain surgery).

July 19th 2002: I was transferred back to Hurstwood Park Neurological Hospital for the Craniotomy, where my Neurosurgeon – Mr Critchley – explained the seriousness of the brain surgery, and the possibilities of my paralysis being increased – 11 hours in the operating theatre (taken apart and rebuilt), 5 titanium plates screwed into my skull and 55 staples to hold it all together, into ICU for 4 days where I suffered 2 post-op Epileptic seizures, and then onto ward for a further 2 weeks…then, at last I was allowed home – able to walk a few paces with a foot brace and stick, but still no use in my arm, and still requiring the use of a wheelchair, but I was alive, I'd beaten the odds, and I was going home.

August 2004: things are looking good, I have been given the 'all clear' from both my neuro-surgeon and rehab consultant, my driving licence has been reinstated (with restrictions), and I'm defying all the original medical predictions – after many, many hours in my local gymnasium, plus privately funded physiotherapy and hydrotherapy, on a good day I can walk over 2 miles without a stick or ankle support, and I have some semi functional use returning in my arm. The downside of my recovery is that my HGV licence and Dangerous Goods certificate have both been revoked by the DVLA for life, which means that I'll never be able to return to my pre-illness employment. Although I've been told that returning to physical work is unlikely, and with short term memory problems and epilepsy, retraining in a different environment would be very difficult, my ultimate goal is to prove them wrong.

February 2005: Despite having to make a 200 mile round trip, I have started Functional Electrical Stimulation treatment at Odstock Hospital, Salisbury, Wiltshire (salisburyfes.com). This treatment has had such a dramatic effect, and improvement on my stability, balance and walking pattern, that I have been able to upgrade my old fitness regime – still 7 days a week / 52 weeks a year – my new daily regime now consists of a 90 minute workout in the gym, followed by a SIX MILE walk (not bad for someone they said was destined never to walk again!) plus hydrotherapy twice a week. Even though I thought that I'd never be able to fly or enjoy a beach holiday again, with the support of my wife, we have had holidays in Malta in 2003, the Dominican Republic in 2004 and Mexico in 2005, and we're now busy planning our next holiday to Canada for 2006, and 'somewhere special' for 2007 (our 25th wedding anniversary).

Unfortunately, many of your family, friends, and work colleagues will let you down, but the ones that don't are your true friends, and they are the ones that will always be there to support both you and your family throughout your recovery – however long it takes.

Just remember, we all have bad days, but the word CAN'T should not be part of your vocabulary – if you really want it, you CAN achieve it.

Jim Shield, 50

Everything seemed to be going without any problem, married with a daughter age 9, house all paid for and a good job. Looking forward to my retirement without a care in the world. Boy was that about to change without any warning.

My 'brain insult' began on Saturday 15th November 2003. I had been busy that day at home making some wardrobe doors for our bedroom, later that day when sitting down I said to my wife that I was having trouble raising my left arm but put this down to too much work on the wardrobe doors.

On the following Monday I went to see my GP who said she would make an appointment at the hospital for me, 'allow up to six weeks' I was told. The following Friday I returned to my GP and was sent to the hospital with a covering letter. I now know that this should have been a blue light job from day one, but before this problem I knew nothing at all about strokes.

In the hospital I had around six hours' wait before getting to see the Doctor, what happened to the urgency of my problem?

The Doctors eventually admitted me into a general ward with not much explanation of what was happening. The first night the patient in the next bed passed away, that did not do much for my much stressed mind, was I next!

It was on the following day that a friendly physiotherapist sat down with me and explained what was going on. I had a mass of questions to be answered: 'what is a stroke?' and most importantly 'why me?'

The stroke had denied me the use of my left side, but never mind, I felt sure this was only a minor thing and I would be well over it in a couple of days! How wrong I was, struggling to make use of my left leg and arm were to become a long running problem.

Eventually I was transferred onto a stroke ward and underwent a barrage of tests. Starting physiotherapy hit home to me just how little I could do. My speech was hit a little and swallowing was a problem, but things which at a push I could live with, but not so the arm and leg which would continue to be big problems.

After a week it began hitting home to me that this was not going to be sorted out by a few exercises. I was then subjected to massive mood swings, laughing and crying for little or no reason and feeling very much alone in the world anxiously wanting to know what tomorrow would bring or indeed if there was going to be a tomorrow.

My wife Sadie came to visit me each day, she always had a smile, but I could see my problem was taking its toll on her life too. She was very supportive, but it was worrying for her seeing me getting weaker each day during the first week.

After three weeks in hospital they set me free, what a wonderful feeling to sleep in your own bed again! I was at home but things would have to change, the little tasks like personal hygiene had become major problems but there are ways to get around things and I was determined to find them. I had quite a few slips on the floor, on the stairs and in the bath, frightened the life out of myself but I had a go.

Soon I discovered what could be done with one hand, even had a go at using a saw to cut wood (and myself). Holding the wood with my good hand and the saw pressed into my tummy, I found that this sort of worked, but the blood on my hands said it was not really a good idea! I found that I could bash a nail in if it was first sat in blue tack to hold the thing in position! Luckily Sadie was willing to lend a hand both with tools and plasters.

At first being at home away from work was ideal as I had all the time in the world to do what I wanted, the trouble was that I couldn't do all I wanted! Yes the Physio had given me a list of exercises to do but progress was painfully slow and I was getting very frustrated with my body not doing what I wanted.

Following advice from my GP I went along to some stroke clubs to be amongst others with similar problems, the first one was a decent drive away (thank God my wife drives) in Suffolk. The club was very friendly with lots to do but they did not allow partners to join which meant my wife was walking around the shops for a couple of hours spending lots of money – not that she seemed to mind that!

The next stroke club which I tried was in my home county of Essex. When we found where the meetings were held we were both disappointed to find most of the patrons looked like they were the wrong side of 100, but they were a friendly lot! They offered us some raffle tickets which we went along with, and when they had the raffle we were well taken back with the prizes – some dusters, a can of hair spray with the top missing and a tired old picture which nobody would bother to pick up if it were dropped onto the floor.

I now attend two stroke clubs, visiting the one in Suffolk every couple of weeks and another one near me which has quite a lot going for it. Still not sure if I entirely accept that I have the same problems as the others, it is very hard to look into the mirror and get a true image of today's me, rather than what I perceive myself to look like.

Although walking is hard work and frustratingly slow I have managed to get myself to the train station to see and have a drink with my workmates. It is even harder sticking to only one alcoholic drink, any more than that and I fall over. Yes, more change!

In order to get me thinking a little more positively about my plight I was advised to attend a course run by the NHS called the Expert Patient Programme. This course ran for one day a week for six weeks and encouraged the likes of me to start thinking positively, set attainable weekly targets and most of all get off your backside and do something! They also covered things like where to go for help and advice should you need it. As I cannot see myself returning to paid work for a good while I have put my name down as a volunteer training assistant for this course and hopefully will be able to spend some time helping others.

I have now got my driving licence back from the DVLA which now allows me to drive an adapted automatic car (but no longer a steam engine!) and have started taking driving lessons on an adapted car driving with one hand (scary). But freedom at last! Watch out you lot I will soon be back on the road!

Next month my present employer will stop my sick pay (half pay) and I have no idea of what will happen then, early retirement perhaps. I would not be able to cope with my old job; the pressures would be too great. My short term memory is far from wonderful, I can't hold a pen to write, have trouble getting some words out and have trouble getting around. But I can use a keyboard with one hand and am determined to do something. The trouble is going to be finding a suitable slot in this big world. After all I am not that old, or am I?

Ruth Clark, 54

I was very fit prior to having my stroke – I worked full time as a nurse, working 7 nights on and 7 off, going to the gym 3 times a week and swimming at least 5 miles a week. I had more energy than people 30 years younger. I went on holiday 3 or 4 times a year; I always kept busy doing something, if the weather was good I would drive out to the countryside and go for a long walk on the moors. I also enjoyed fell walking rain or shine. At first I could not believe it had happened to me, as I was so fit. The doctors told me that if I had not been fit I would not have survived and there were many times I wish I hadn't. I am now glad that I did as I now have 3 grandchildren. I wanted to be a proper hands-on granny; baby-sitting and every thing, now I cannot even pick them up.

I now live independently with the help of carers. I have been to college and done a GCSE course in psychology but failed the exam due to my memory problems. I have also learnt to swim. Sometimes I am so angry about it as I was planning my retirement. I had planned to buy a small bungalow and do voluntary work for a couple of years or go backpacking around the world. As I used to live in a 2nd floor flat I had to move and have quite a nice ground floor flat now.

Useful Addresses

Please remember that addresses and contact information can change with time. There are numerous groups giving information on stroke that may be of help to you or other interested parties. These include groups that exist to help people quit smoking and to provide guidance on reducing salt and alcohol consumption. I have not included the contact details for these groups here. These will be available from doctors' surgeries, government offices, local libraries and citizens' advice centres. I have chosen to provide what I consider to be useful contact details by country, under the following headings:

- Stroke

- Financial

- Head and brain injury

- Movement and mobility

- Physiotherapy

- Speech and language

- Care

- Counselling

Australia

Stroke

National Stroke Foundation
Level 3, 167–169 Queen Street
Melbourne, VIC 3000
Tel: 03 9670 1000 Fax: 03 9670 9300
www.strokefoundation.com.au

Financial

Australian Federation of Disability Organisations
Ross House, 247 Flinders Lane
Melbourne, VIC 3000
Tel: 03 9662 3324 Fax: 03 9662 3325
www.disfed.org.au

Australian Institute of Health and Welfare
GPO Box 570
Canberra, ACT 2601
Tel: 02 6244 1000 Fax: 02 6244 1299
www.aihw.gov.au

Department of Families and Community Services
Box 7788, Canberra Mail Centre
Canberra, ACT 2610
Tel: 1300 653 227 (Toll Free)
www.facs.gov.au

Heart Support Australia
PO Box 266
Mawson, ACT 2607
Tel: 02 6285 2357 Fax: 02 6281 1120
www.heartnet.org.au

National Council on Intellectual Disability
PO Box 771
Mawson, ACT 2607
Tel: 02 6296 4400 Fax: 02 6296 4488
www.dice.org.au

National Ethnic Disability Alliance
PO Box 381
Harris Park, NSW 2150
Tel: 1800 629 072 (Toll Free)
Fax: 02 9635 5355
www.neda.org.au

Women With Disabilities (Australia)
PO Box 605
Rosny Park, TAS 7018
Tel: 03 6244 8288 Fax: 03 6244 8255
www.wwda.org.au

Head and brain injury

Acquired Brain Injury Service
Arbias
PO Box 213
Fitzroy, VIC 3065
Tel: 03 9417 7071 Fax: 03 9417 7056
www.arbias.org.au

Brain Injury Australia
PO Box 82
Mawson, ACT 2607
Tel: 02 6290 2253 Fax: 02 6290 2252
www.braininjuryaustralia.com.au

Movement and mobility

Physical Disability Council of Australia
PO Box 77
Northgate, QLD 4013
Tel: 07 3267 1057 Fax: 07 3267 1733
www.pdca.org.au

Physiotherapy

Australian Physiotherapy Association
Level 3, 201 Fitzroy Street
St. Kilda
Melbourne, VIC 182
Tel: 03 9534 9400 Fax: 03 9534 9199
www.physiotherapy.asn.au

Commonwealth Rehabilitation Service (CRS Australia)
25 Argyle Street
Hobart, TAS 7000
Tel: 1800 624 824 (Toll Free)
www.crsrehab.gov.au

Speech and language

Speech Pathology Australia
2nd Floor, 11–19 Bank Place
Melbourne, VIC 3000
Tel: 03 9642 4899 Fax: 03 9642 4922
www.speechpathologyaustralia.org.au

Care

Carers Australia
PO Box 73
Deakin West, ACT 2600
Tel: 02 6122 9900 Fax: 02 6122 9999
www.carersaustralia.com.au

Carers Association of South Australia
58 King William Road
Goodwood, SA 5034
Tel: 1800 815 549 (Toll Free)
Fax: 08 8271 6388
www.carers-sa.asn.au

Counselling

Anxiety Treatment Australia
Floor 1, 140–142 Barkers Road
Hawthorn, VIC 3122
Tel: 03 9819 3671
www.anxietyaustralia.com.au

Australian Counselling Association
PO Box 33
Kedron, QLD 4031
Tel: 07 3857 8288 Fax: 07 3857 1777
www.theaca.net.au

Lifeline Australia National Office
PO Box 173
Deakin, ACT 2600
Tel: 02 6215 9400 Fax: 02 6282 6566
www.lifeline.org.au

Canada

Stroke

Heart and Stroke Foundation of Canada
222 Queen Street, Suite 1402
Ottawa, ON K1P 5V9
Tel: 613 569 4361 Fax: 613 569 3278
www.heartandstroke.ca

Financial

Government of Canada
Office for Disability Issues
300 Laurier Avenue West
Ottawa, ON K1A 0J6
Tel: 1800 622 6232 (Toll Free)
www.sdc.gc.ca/en/gateways/nav/top_nav/pr
ogram/odi.shtml

Head and brain injury

Neurologic Rehabilitation Institute of Ontario
59 Beaver Bend Crescent
Etobicoke, ON M9B 5R2
Tel: 1800 561 9158 (Toll free)
www.nrio.com

Movement and mobility

Active Living Coalition for Older Adults
33 Laird Drive
Toronto, ON M4G 3S9
Tel: 1800 549 9799 (Toll Free)
Fax: 416 423 2112
www.alcoa.ca

Physiotherapy

Canadian Physiotherapy Association
2345 Yonge Street, Suite 410
Toronto, ON M4P 2E5
Tel: 1800 387 8679 (Toll Free)
Fax: 416 932 9708

Speech and language

Canadian Association of Speech-Language Pathologists and Audiologists
401–200 Elgin Street
Ottawa, ON K2P 1L5
Tel: 1800 259 8519 (Toll Free)
Fax: 613 567 2859
www.caslpa.ca

Care

Canadian Homecare Association
17 York Street, Suite 401
Ottawa, ON K1N 9J6
Tel: 613 569 1585 Fax: 613 569 1604
www.cdnhomecare.ca

Counselling

Canadian Counselling Association
116 Albert Street, Suite 702
Ottawa, ON K1P 5G3
Tel: 1877 756 5565 (Toll Free)
Fax: 613 237 9786
www.ccacc.ca

Republic of Ireland

Stroke

Irish Heart Foundation
4 Clyde Road
Ballsbridge
Dublin 4
Tel: 01 668 5001 Fax: 01 668 5896
www.irishheart.ie

Diabetes Federation of Ireland
76 Lower Gardiner Street
Dublin 1
Tel: 01 836 3022 Fax: 01 836 5182
www.diabetes.ie

The Volunteer Stroke Scheme
249 Crumlin Road
Dublin 12
Tel: 01 455 9036 Fax: 01 455 7013

Financial

FAS – Training and Employment Authority (Ireland)
PO Box 456
27–33 Upper Baggot Street
Dublin 4
Tel: 01 607 0500 Fax: 01 607 0600

Head and brain injury

Headway
1–3 Manor Business Park
Manor Street
Dublin 7
Tel: 01 810 2066 Fax: 01 810 2070
Helpline: 1890 200 278
www.headwayireland.ie

Movement and mobility

Irish Wheelchair Association
Áras Chúchulainn
Blackheath Drive
Dublin 3
Tel: 01 833 3884
www.iwa.ie

Physiotherapy

National Rehabilitation Board
Upper Mallow Street
Limerick
Tel: 061 319779 Fax: 061 412977

Speech and language

Irish Association of Speech and Language Therapists
29 Gardiner Place
Dublin 1
Tel: 01 878 0215
www.iaslt.com

Care

The Carers Association
'Prior's Orchard'
John's Quay
Kilkenny
Tel: 056 772 1424 Fax: 056 775 3531
www.carersireland.com/

Counselling

Irish Association for Counselling and Psychotherapy
8 Cumberland Street
Dun Laoghaire
Co. Dublin
Tel: 01 230 0061 Fax: 01 230 0064
www.irish-counselling.ie

United Kingdom

Stroke

The Stroke Association
240 City Road
London EC1V 2PR
Tel: 020 7566 0300
Fax: 020 7490 2686
National Stroke Helpline: 0845 30 33 100
www.stroke.org.uk

The Stroke Association (Wales)
74 Merthyr Road
Whitchurch
Cardiff CF14 1DJ
Tel: 029 20 61 1121
Fax: 029 20 61 1171
www.stroke.org.uk

Chest, Heart and Stroke Scotland
65 North Castle Street
Edinburgh EH2 3LT
Tel: 0131 225 6963
Fax: 0131 220 6313
www.chss.org.uk

Northern Ireland Chest, Heart and Stroke Association
22 Great Victoria Street
Belfast BT2 7LX
Tel: 028 9032 0184
Fax: 028 9033 3487
Advice Helpline: 0845 769 7299 (Lo-Call)
www.nichsa.com

Different Strokes
9 Canon Harnett Court
Wolverton Mill
Milton Keynes MK12 5NF
Tel: 0845 130 7172 (Lo-Call), 01908 317618
Fax: 01908 313501
www.differentstrokes.co.uk

Financial

Disabled Living Foundation
380–384 Harrow Road
London W9 2HU
Tel: 020 7289 6111
www.dlf.org.uk

Employment Opportunities
53 New Broad Street
London EC2M 1SL
Tel: 020 7448 5420
Fax: 020 7374 4913
email: info@eopps.org

Department of Health
Richmond House
79 Whitehall
London SW1A 2NL
Tel: 020 7210 4850
www.dh.gov.uk

Head and brain injury

Brain and Spine Foundation
7 Winchester House
Kennington Park
Cranmer Road
London SW9 6EJ
Tel: 020 7793 5900
www.brainandspine.org.uk

British Neuroscience Association
Sherrington Buildings
Ashton Street
Liverpool L69 3GE
Tel: 0151 794 4943
Fax: 0151 794 5516
www.bna.org.uk

Headway
4 King Edward Court
King Edward Street
Nottingham NG1 1EW
Tel: 0115 924 0800
Fax: 0115 958 4446
www.headway.org.uk

Movement and mobility

Disabled Drivers Association
Ashwellthorpe
Norwich NR16 1AX
Tel: 0870 770 3333
Fax: 01508 488173
www.dda.org.uk

Disabled Living Centres Council
Redbank House
4 St Chad's Street
Manchester M8 8QA
Tel: 0161 834 1044
Fax: 0161 835 3591
www.dlcc.org.uk

HemiHelp
Unit 1, Wellington Works
Wellington Road
London SW19 8EQ
Tel: 0845 120 3713 (Lo-Call)
Fax: 0845 120 3723 (Lo-Call)
www.hemihelp.org.uk

MAVIS (Mobility Advice and Vehicle Information Service)
Crowthorne Business Estate
Old Wokingham Road
Crowthorne RG45 6XD
Tel: 01344 661000 Fax: 01344 661066
www.dft.gov.uk/access/mavis

Motability
City Gate House
22 Southwark Bridge Road
London SE1 9HB
Tel: 0845 456 4566 (Lo-Call)
Fax: 020 7928 1818
www.motability.co.uk

RADAR (Royal Association for Disability and Rehabilitation)
12 City Forum
250 City Road
London EC1V 8AF
Tel: 020 7250 3222 Fax: 020 7250 0212
www.radar.org.uk

Rehab UK
Windermere House
Kendal Avenue
London W3 0XA
Tel: 020 8896 2333
Fax: 020 8896 2444
www.rehabuk.org

Physiotherapy

Chartered Society of Physiotherapy (CSP)
www.csp.org.uk

CSP England
14 Bedford Row
London WC1R 4ED
Tel: 020 7306 6666 Fax: 020 7306 6611

CSP Scotland
21 Queen Street
Edinburgh EH2 1JX
Tel: 0131 226 1441
Fax: 0131 226 1551

CSP Wales
1 Cathedral Road
Cardiff CF11 9SD
Tel/fax: 029 2038 2429

CSP Northern Ireland
Merrion Business Centre
Belfast BT1 6PJ
Tel: 028 9050 1803
Fax: 028 9050 1804

Speech and language

Action for Dysphasic Adults (ADA)
1 Royal Street
London SE1 7LL
Tel: 020 7261 9572
Fax: 020 7928 9542
www.speakability.org.uk

Afasic
2nd Floor, 50–52 Great Sutton Street
London EC1V 0DJ
Tel: 020 7490 9410
Fax: 020 7251 2834
www.afasic.org.uk

Royal College of Speech and Language Therapists
7 Bath Place
Rivington Street
London EC2A 3DR
Tel: 020 7613 3855
Fax: 020 7613 3854
www.rcslt.org

Connect
16–18 Marshalsea Road
Southwark
London SE1 1HL
Tel: 020 7367 0840
Fax: 020 7367 0841
www.ukconnect.org

Care

Association of Independent Care Advisers
Orchard House
Albury
Surrey GU5 9AG
Tel: 01483 203066
Fax: 01483 202535
www.aica.org.uk

Carers UK
20–25 Glasshouse Yard
London EC1A 4JT
Tel: 020 7490 8818
Fax: 020 7490 8824
www.carersuk.org

Crossroads Association
10 Regent Place
Rugby
Warwickshire CV21 2PN
Tel: 0845 450 0350 (Lo-Call)
Fax: 01788 565498
www.crossroads.org.uk

Registered Nursing Homes Association
15 Highfield Road
Edgbaston
Birmingham B15 3DU
Tel: 0121 454 2511
Fax: 0121 454 9032
www.rnha.co.uk

National Council for Voluntary Organisations
Regent's Wharf
8 All Saints Street
London N1 9RL
Tel: 0800 2 798 798 (Freefone)
Fax: 020 7713 6300
www.ncvo-vol.org.uk

United Kingdom Homecare Association
42b Banstead Road
Carshalton Beeches
Surrey SM5 3NW
Tel: 020 8288 1551
Fax: 020 8288 1550
www.ukhca.co.uk

Counselling

British Association for Counselling and Psychotherapy
BACP House
35–37 Albert Street
Rugby
Warwickshire CV21 2SG
Tel: 0870 443 5252
Fax: 0870 443 5161
www.bacp.co.uk

Clinical hypnotherapy

BST Foundation
5 Kingsholm House
106 Ridgeway
Wimbledon
London SW1 4RD
Tel: 020 8946 1432
www.bstfoundation.co.uk

USA

Stroke

American Stroke Association
7272 Greenville Avenue
Dallas, TX 75231
Tel: 800 242 1871 (Toll Free)
Fax: 214 570 5930
www.strokeassociation.org

American Council for Headache Education
19 Mantua Road
Mt. Royal, NJ 08061
Tel: 856 423 0258 Fax: 856 423 0082
www.achenet.org

Brain Aneurysm Foundation
12 Clarendon Street
Boston, MA 0211
Tel: 617 723 3870 Fax: 617 723 8672
www.bafound.org

Children's Hemiplegia and Stroke Association
4101 West Green Oaks Boulevard, Suite 305
PMB 149
Arlington, TX 76016
Tel: 817 492 4325
www.chasa.org

Hazel K. Goddess Fund for Stroke Research in Women
785 Park Avenue
New York, NY 10021-3552
Tel: 212 734 8067 Fax: 212 288 2160
www.thegoddessfund.org

National Aphasia Association
PO Box 1887
Murray Hill Station
New York, NY 10156
Tel: 800 922 4622 (Toll Free)
Fax: 212 267 2812
www.aphasia.org

National Heart, Lung and Blood Institute
PO Box 30105
Bethesda, MD 20824-0105
Tel: 301 592 8573 Fax: 240 629 3246
www.nhlbi.nih.gov

National Institute of Neurological Disorders and Stroke
Neurological Institute
PO Box 5801
Bethesda, MD 20824
Tel: 301 496 5751
www.ninds.nih.gov

National Stroke Association
9707 East Easter Lane
Englewood, CO 80112
Tel: 800 787 6537 (Toll Free)
Fax: 303 649 1328
www.stroke.org

Financial

American Health Assistance Foundation
22512 Gateway Center Drive
Clarksburg, MD 20871
Tel: 301 948 3244 Fax: 301 258 9454
www.ahaf.org

Heart Support of America
6344 Clinton Highway
Knoxville, TN 37912
Tel: 865 938 5838
Fax: 865 938 6096
www.heartsupport.com

US Department of Labor
Frances Perkins Building
200 Constitution Avenue, NW
Washington, DC 20210
Tel: 866 633 7365 (Toll Free)
Fax: 202 693 7888
www.dol.gov/odep

National Council on the Aging
300 D Street SW, Suite 801
Washington, DC 20024
Tel: 202 479 1200 Fax: 202 479 0735
www.ncoa.org

Head and brain injury

Brain Injury Association of America
8201 Greensboro Drive, Suite 611
McLean, VA 22102
Tel: 703 761 0750 Fax: 703 761 0755
www.biausa.org

Movement and mobility

American Occupational Therapy Association
4720 Montgomery Lane
PO Box 31220
Bethesda, MD 20824-1220
Tel: 301 652 2682 Fax: 301 652 7711
www.aota.org

Association for Driver Rehabilitation Specialists
711 S. Vienna Street
Ruston, LA 71270
Tel: 800 290 2344 (Toll Free)
Fax: 318 255 4175
www.driver-ed.org

Physiotherapy

American Physical Therapy Association
1111 North Fairfax Street
Alexandria, VA 22314-1488
Tel: 800 999 2782 Fax: 703 684 7343
www.apta.org

National Rehabilitation Information Center
4200 Forbes Boulevard, Suite 202
Lanham, MD 20706-4829
Tel: 301 459 5900 Fax: 301 562 2401
www.naric.com

Speech and language

American Speech-Language-Hearing Association
10801 Rockville Pike
Rockville, MD 20852
Tel: 800 638 8255 (Toll Free)
Fax: 301 571 0457
www.asha.org

Care

National Family Caregivers Association
10400 Connecticut Avenue, Suite 500
Kensington, MD 20895-3944
Tel: 800 896 3650 (Toll Free)
Fax: 301 942 2302
www.thefamilycaregiver.org

The Well Spouse Foundation
63 West Main Street, Suite H
Freehold, NJ 07728
Tel: 800 838 0879 (Toll Free)
Fax: 732 577 8899
www.wellspouse.org

Counselling

Job Accommodation Network
PO Box 6080
Morgantown, WV 26506-6080
Tel: 800 526 7234 (Toll Free)
Fax: 304 293 5407
http://janweb.icdi.wvu.e

Glossary

Acquired brain injury is one that is not congenital, meaning that it occurred at a specific time after birth. Acquired brain injury may be the result of physical trauma or various medical conditions.

Acute Medical Units have a fast track system for patients referred by GPs or the accident and emergency department that helps reduce the number of patients admitted to hospital and helps shorten the hospital stay of those who are admitted.

Adrenaline is a natural stimulant. It is one of two chemicals (the other is norepinephrine) released by the adrenal gland that increases the speed and force of heart beats. It dilates the airways to improve breathing and narrows blood vessels in the skin and intestine so that an increased flow of blood reaches the muscles and allows them to cope with stress or the demands of exercise.

Agnosia is the ability to recognise objects by using the senses (or a given sense) even though the senses (or the sense used) remain undamaged. The term is derived from the Greek meaning 'lack of knowledge'.

Agraphia is the inability to write properly.

Alexia is an acquired impairment in the ability to comprehend written words. The disorder is often quite specific in that sufferers do not have impairment of vision and can identify spoken words normally.

Alzheimer's disease is a degenerative disease of the brain (dementia) in which the person gradually loses cognitive functioning.

Aneurysm is a blood-filled sac caused by the swelling of the wall of a blood vessel.

Anomia is the inability to name objects.

Anoxia is a lack of oxygen.

Antiemetics are a group of medications used to decrease or control nausea and vomiting.

Aphasia is a difficulty in understanding and using spoken or written language. It is, in effect, an absence of language. While it is more serious than dysphasia the two terms are often used interchangeably.

Aphemia is the loss of the power of speaking, while retaining the power of writing.

Aphonia is the inability to naturally produce speech sounds that require the use of the larynx that is not due to a lesion in the central nervous system.

Apoplexy is a sudden loss of consciousness resulting when the rupture or occlusion of a blood vessel leads to oxygen lack in the brain. It is generally used interchangeably with the terms stroke, cerebrovascular accident (CVA) and brain attack.

Apraxia is a motor-planning disability. It is the inability to do complex tasks when requested even though there is no paralysis of the muscles. It may refer to motor planning, movement or to speech and language functions. In terms of the latter, it is a term used interchangeably with dyspraxia. Apraxia may affect almost any voluntary movements, including those required for proper eye gaze, walking, speaking or writing.

Arteriosclerosis is a general term for various disorders of the arteries. It is a chronic disease in which thickening, hardening and loss of elasticity of the arterial walls result in impaired blood circulation. It develops primarily with ageing, and often as the result of hypertension and diabetes.

Ataxia is a lack of motor co-ordination due to irregularities in timing, rate and force of muscular contraction.

Atherosclerosis is a condition in which the arteries become blocked with plaques.

Atrial fibrillation is a heartbeat irregularity causing blood clots to form in the heart itself.

Blood pressure is the pressure of the blood against the inner walls of the arteries. It is measured in millimetres of mercury and is given as two readings: systolic blood pressure is the top number and reflects the pressure in the arteries when the heart is pumping; diastolic blood pressure is the bottom number and represents the arterial pressure when the heart is resting. Normal blood pressure is 120/80.

Blood sugar tests are done primarily to test for diabetes.

Brain attack is a term used interchangeably with stroke or cerebrovascular accident (CVA). It happens when brain cells die because of inadequate blood flow to the brain.

Cardiomyopathy is a disease of the heart muscle that causes it to lose its pumping strength. There can be many causes.

Carotid artery dissection (CAD) is a dissection or tear in the carotid artery that can divert blood flow and cause constriction of the artery. It is increasingly recognised as a cause of stroke in younger patients.

Carotid artery ultrasound scan is an imaging procedure that uses high-frequency soundwaves to view the blood vessels in the neck to determine the presence of narrowing in the carotid arteries.

Carotid endarterectomy is the surgical removal of plaque that is blocking or reducing blood flow in a carotid artery.

Cerebral embolism is a blood clot in the brain that originates from elsewhere in the body.

Cerebral oedema is a swelling in brain tissue caused by irritation from bleeding.

Cerebrovascular disease is any disease affecting an artery within the brain, or supplying blood to the brain.

Cervical artery dissection is a dissection or tear in a cervical artery (carotid and vertebral arteries).

Cervical laminectomy is a surgical intervention performed on the cervical (neck) vertebrae.

Cholesterol is a soft, waxy substance found among the lipids (fats) in the bloodstream and in all the body's cells.

Chorea is an involuntary abrupt, rapid, brief and unsustained irregular movement.

Colour agnosia is a difficulty in identifying colours.

Congenital heart disease is a heart defect or condition present at birth.

Cortisol is the body's natural stress-fighting and anti-inflammatory hormone.

Cranial nerves control the sensory and muscle functions around the eyes, face and throat.

CT (computed tomography) brain scan produces pictures of structures within the body. Images are created by a computer that takes the data from multiple X-ray images and turns them into pictures on a screen.

Depersonalisation is such a change in an individual's self-awareness that they feel detached from their own experience, with the self, the body and mind seeming alien.

Derealisation is a feeling of disconnection from the world around. It is a dreamlike state.

Diabetes is a condition in which the body either cannot produce insulin or cannot effectively use the insulin it produces.

Diplopia is the medical term for double vision.

Disability Adjusted Life Years is a summary measure that combines the impact of illness, disability and mortality on population health.

Dissociation is a mental response that diverts consciousness from painful or traumatic events.

Dopamine is a neurotransmitter, or chemical, that transmits signals between nerve cells. It is present in regions of the brain that regulate movement, emotion, motivation and the feeling of pleasure.

Dysarthria is the inability to articulate clearly due to facial paralysis, which can produce weaknesses and co-ordination difficulties to the muscles of the face, tongue and throat. It can result from a stroke occurring in any one of several parts of the brain.

Dyscalculia refers to a difficulty with mathematics.

Dysdiadochokinesia is the inability to perform rapidly alternating movements.

Dysmetria is the 'overshoot' or 'undershoot' of a reaching movement.

Dysphagia is the term used to describe a difficulty in swallowing.

Dysphasia is a dysfunction of language. It is a term used interchangeably with aphasia to cover a variety of language problems.

Dysphonia is the impaired ability to produce sound.

Dyspraxia is a difficulty in performing complex tasks like articulation, consciously. It is a term used interchangeably with apraxia.

Dysrhymokinesis refers to a disrupted rhythm of fine motor movements, e.g. finger or foot tapping.

Dyssynergia is an inability to smoothly perform the elements of a movement in the appropriate space and the correct time, and errors in the speed and sequence of the component parts of a movement causes a breakdown of a multi-joint movement into its constituent parts.

Echocardiogram is a non-invasive test that uses soundwaves to produce a study of the motion of the heart's chambers and valves. The echo soundwaves create an image on the monitor as an ultrasound transducer is passed over the heart. The soundwaves are bounced off the walls and chambers of the heart, allowing the heart's shape and motion, as well as the presence of clots, to be seen and measured.

Electrocardiogram (ECG) is a graphic tracing of the heart's electrical activity, used in diagnosing some heart abnormalities.

Embolic stroke occurs when a blood clot originating from elsewhere in the body travels to the brain and becomes wedged in a vessel that supplies blood to the brain.

Endocrinologists diagnose and treat conditions of the endocrine system (glands and hormones).

Endorphins are biochemical substances made by the body that may help reduce pain and may contribute to positive moods.

Glucose is a form of sugar that is the body's primary fuel; glucose broken down from food can be converted into energy or stored. Abnormally low or high levels of glucose in the blood often indicate metabolic disturbances (e.g. diabetes).

Glycemic index is a measure of the rate at which foods break down and enter the bloodstream as glucose.

Grey matter is the tissue of the nervous system that appears grey because of the relatively high proportion of nerve cell nuclei that occur there.

Haemorrhagic stroke occurs when a blood vessel in the brain bursts, spilling blood into the spaces surrounding the brain cells, or when a cerebral aneurysm ruptures. It is also called an intracranial haemorrhage.

Heart rate is the number of heartbeats in a minute.

Hemianaesthesia is a lack of feeling and position on one side of the body.

Hemianopsia is defective vision or blindness in half of one or both eyes.

Hemiparesis is a weakness on one side of the body.

Hemiplegia is paralysis on one side of the body.

High-density lipoprotein (HDL) is a particle in the blood. HDL is known as 'good' cholesterol because it deposits cholesterol in the liver, where it is then excreted by the body. High HDL is thought to protect against coronary artery disease.

Hormones are proteins produced by the endocrine glands of the body that trigger activity in other locations.

Hydrocephalus is an excessive amount of cerebrospinal fluid usually under increased pressure within the skull. The condition may be congenital, result from a head injury, brain haemorrhage, infection or tumour. It is sometimes the first sign of spina bifida or can be caused by surgery to close an open spinal column.

Hypercholesterolaemia is the presence of high levels of cholesterol in the blood. It is not a disease but a metabolic state that can be secondary to many diseases and can contribute to many forms of disease, most notably cardiovascular disease.

Hyperglycemia is abnormally high levels of glucose in the blood.

Hyperkinesia is too much movement.

Hyperventilation is rapid, shallow and erratic breathing.

Hypokinesia is too little movement.

Hypoperfusion is a reduction in overall blood flow to an organ (in the case of the brain this is generally due to a build-up of atherosclerotic plaque).

Hypotonia is the defective maintenance of posture.

Infarct is an area of cell death (e.g. part of the brain) as a result of being deprived of its blood, and consequently its oxygen, supply.

Insulin is a hormone produced by the pancreas, which is necessary for glucose to be able to enter the cells of the body and be used for energy.

Intracerebral haemorrhage is a bleed that occurs within the brain itself.

Ischaemic cascade is the chemical chain reaction resulting from brain cell death.

Ischaemic stroke is a stroke caused by a blockage of an artery or blood vessel, which interrupts blood flow to the brain. This is the most common category (by cause) of stroke and is also called a cerebral infarction.

Lactulose is a non-absorbable synthetic sugar, which is used as a cathartic (laxative) to treat chronic constipation and disturbances of function in the central nervous system.

Laminectomy is an operation for removal of part or all of the lamina of a vertebra.

Laxative is a substance that promotes bowel movements.

Life coach is someone trained to help with 'whole-life dilemmas' (e.g. personal relationships, work–life balance) or with career development (e.g. stress burn-out, finance, critical thinking).

Low-density lipoprotein (LDL) is the type of protein particle that carries lipids in the blood and allows the fat to be deposited into the walls of arteries. LDL is the 'bad' cholesterol when measured in a blood test.

Lumbar puncture (spinal tap) tests drain a small sample of cerebral spinal fluid from the lower spine. A needle is inserted between the vertebrae (backbones) in the lower back and into the space containing the spinal fluid.

Magnetic resonance imaging (MRI) is an imaging technique that uses radio waves, magnetic fields, and computer analysis to provide a picture of body tissues and structures.

Movement agnosia is the inability to recognise the movement of an object.

Neurones are nerve cells.

Neuroplasticity is the brain's ability, at the level of the neurone, to recover structurally and/or functionally after injury or disease.

Norepinephrine is a neurotransmitter found mainly in areas of the brain that are involved in governing autonomic nervous system activity, such as blood pressure and heart rate.

Nystagmus refers to rapid involuntary movements of the eyes that may be from side to side, up and down, or rotary. Depending on the cause, these movements may be in both eyes or in just one eye.

Ocular dysynergia is a failure of either eye to move promptly, or smoothly. It is best tested by asking the patient to follow the slow movement of a visual target across the visual field.

Ophthalmoscope is a lighted instrument used to examine the inside of the eye, including the retina and the optic nerve.

Oral glucose tolerance test is a test to diagnose borderline diabetes and early diabetes. The test requires fasting overnight, then drinking a high-glucose beverage. Blood samples are taken every hour for several hours to see how well the body uses sugar.

Oxygen saturation is the extent to which the haemoglobin is saturated with oxygen. Haemoglobin is an element in the bloodstream that binds with oxygen and carries it to the organs and tissues of the body. A normal oxygen saturation of the blood leaving the heart to the body is 95 to 100 per cent, while the oxygen saturation of the blood returning to the heart after delivering oxygen to the body is 75 per cent.

Parasympathetic nervous system originates in the brainstem and lower part of the spinal cord. It is primarily aroused in states of rest and relaxation and opposes the physiological effects of the sympathetic nervous system. It conserves energy as it slows the heart, lowers blood pressure, slows the rate of breathing, constricts the pupils, dilates blood vessels, increases intestinal and gland activity, and relaxes sphincter muscles.

Penumbra is an area of stroke-damaged, oxygen-starved tissue surrounding the infarct that is not irretrievably injured.

Percutaneous transluminal angioplasty is also known as balloon angioplasty. It involves stretching and widening a narrowed artery.

Pericardial infusion is when there is a fluid around the heart.

Phlebotomist is a person who takes blood specimens from people's veins.

Polycarbophil restores normal moisture levels to the intestine and helps produce well-formed stools. It is used to treat certain types of diarrhoea or constipation.

Prosopagnosia is the selective inability to recognise the faces of familiar people.

Psyllium is a soluble fibre, often labelled as a laxative, that comes from a plant most commonly grown in India. It is not absorbed in the small bowel. It is broken down in the large bowel and becomes a food source for the bacteria that live in the colon. These healthy bacteria bulk up the stool, creating a larger, softer stool, which is easier to pass.

Quadriparesis is a severe or complete loss of motor function in all four limbs.

Reflexologists work with the body's energy flow to stimulate self-healing by manipulating 'reflex' areas of the body (feet, hands, ears) that correspond to other parts of the body.

Saturated fats are among the most common fats in our diet. They are found predominantly in animal foods like meat, poultry and full-fat dairy products, and in tropical oils like palm and coconut. Diets high in saturated fats are associated with higher risks of heart disease, certain cancers, and stroke.

Scanning speech is slurred speech after a stroke.

Simvastatin is a substance used to reduce the amount of cholesterol and certain fatty substances in the blood.

Sphygmomanometers are used to measure blood pressure.

Stroke belt is the southeast area of the USA identified as contributing a statistical anomaly by having a high stroke rate. It is made up of 11 states (Alabama, Arkansas, Georgia, Indiana, Kentucky, Louisiana, Mississippi, North Carolina, South Carolina, Tennessee, and Virginia).

Subarachnoid haemorrhage is a bleed in the space between the brain and the skull.

Sympathetic nervous system originates in the thoracic regions of the spinal cord. It is the part of the nervous system over which a person does not have conscious control (e.g. glands, heart, blood vessels and smooth muscle).

Thrombotic stroke occurs when a blood clot blocks a vessel that supplies blood to the brain.

Thromboxane is a substance that causes blood clotting and constriction of blood vessels.

Transient ischaemic attack is a period of disturbance of body function, lasting for less than 24 hours, resulting from a temporary reduction in blood supply to part of the brain.

Transoesophageal echocardiogram is used to obtain a more clear two-dimensional echocardiogram of the heart.

Triglyceride is a fat found in the blood. Most fat found in the diet and body is in the form of triglycerides. Excess triglycerides are stored in adipose tissue and are used to provide energy. Elevated blood levels of triglycerides and of cholesterol may be associated with an increased risk for atherosclerosis and related disorders, such as coronary artery disease, heart attack and hypertension.

Truncal ataxia is a syndrome displayed when a person is unable to sit on their bed without steadying themselves.

Vascular dementia is a group of disorders in which brain cells are damaged by abnormal blood circulation to the brain.

Vertebral artery dissection (VAD) is a dissection or tear in the vertebral artery that can divert blood flow and cause constriction of the artery. It is increasingly recognised as a cause of stroke in younger patients.

Vertigo is defined as an affliction of the head in which objects, though stationary, appear to move in various directions, and the person affected finds it difficult to maintain an erect posture. It is often accompanied by nausea and occasionally vomiting, and is generally worsened by motion. Sometimes caused by blood vessel compression of balance nerves.

White matter is the tissue of the nervous system that consists mainly of axons. It is white because of the insulating lipid-protein sheath found around the axons.

World Health Organization (WHO) is an agency of the United Nations, acting as a co-ordinating authority on international public health, headquartered in Geneva, Switzerland. The WHO was established by the United Nations on 7 April 1948.

References

Altschuler, E.L., Wisdom, S.B., Stone, L., Foster, C., Galaska, D., Llewellyn, D.M. and Ramachandran, V.S. (1999) 'Rehabilitation of hemiparesis after stroke with a mirror.' *Lancet 353*, 2035–2036.

Berk, L. (1989) 'Neuroendocrine influences of mirthful laughter.' *American Journal of Medical Sciences 298*, 390–396.

Carroll, R.T. (2003) *The Sceptic's Dictionary*. Chichester: Wiley.

Ditty, W. (2001) *One Brain – Two Halves*. www.bbc.co.uk/dna/hzgz/alabaster/ A659874.

Ellis, A., Wiseman, W. and Boss, K. (1991) *Fundamentals of Chinese Acupuncture*. Brookline, MA: Paradigm Publications.

Gordon, N., Gulanick, M., Costa, F., Fletcher, G., Franklin, B., Roth, E. and Sheppard, T. (2004) 'Physical activity and exercise recommendations for stroke survivors.' *Circulation 109*, 2031–2041.

Grant, N. (1994) *Laurel & Hardy: Quote Unquote*. Bath: Parragon.

Hachinski, V. and Hachinski, L. (2004) *'The Daily Telegraph' Stroke: What You Really Need to Know*. London: Constable and Robinson.

Hinds, D.M. (2000) *After Stroke*. London: Thorsons.

Jacobson, E. (1974) *Progressive Relaxation: A Physiological and Clinical Investigation of Muscular States and their Significance in Psychology and Medical Practice*. Chicago: University of Chicago Press. (Originally published 1929.)

Jonas, B. and Mussolino, M.E. (2000) 'Symptoms of depression as a prospective risk factor for stroke.' *Psychosomatic Medicine 62*, 463–471.

Keys, A. (1970) 'Coronary heart disease in seven countries.' *Circulation 41* (Suppl 1), 1–211.

Lamontagne, A. and Fung, J. (2004) 'Faster is better: Implications for speed-intensive gait training after stroke.' *Stroke 35*, 2543–2548.

Lantin, B. (2003) 'Fatigue after Stroke.' *Stroke News 21.4*, 22–23.

Lehr Jr., R.P. (1998) 'Brain Functions and Brain Map.' Presentation paper. Department of Anatomy, School of Medicine, Southern Illinois University, Springfield, IL.

McLaren, B. (2004) *The Voice of Rugby: My Autobiography*. London: Bantam Press.

Murray, M.W. (2004) 'Heart Disease: Tips for Prevention.' www.umm.edu/features/tips_prev.html

Stroke Association (2004) 'Balance problems explained.' *Stroke News 22.2*, 20–21.

Szegedi, A., Kohnen, R., Dienel, A. and Kieser, M. (2005) 'Acute treatment of moderate to severe depression with hypericum extract WS 5570 (St John's wort): Randomised controlled double blind non-inferiority trial versus paroxetin.' *British Medical Journal 330*, 503.

Taycan, O., Uyankik, O., Tanriverdi, T., Ertan, S. and Kiziltan, G. (2002) 'Can cerebellar infarctions be overlooked?' *Journal of Neurological Studies 20*, 1, 51–55.

Wiebers, D. (2001) *Stroke Free For Life: The Complete Guide to Stroke Prevention and Treatment.* London: Vermilion.

Wiseman, R. (2004) *Did You Spot the Gorilla? How to Recognise Hidden Opportunities.* London: Arrow Books.

Further Reading

Berkowitz, D., Wolkowitz, B., Fitch, R. and Kopriva, R. (2000) *The Use of Tests as Part of High-Stakes Decision-Making for Students: A Resources Guide for Educators and Policy-Makers.* Washington, DC: US Department of Education.

Bestic, L. (2004) 'Coping with change.' *Stroke News 22*, 1, 16–17.

Bradford, N. (1995) *Men's Health Matters: The Complete A–Z of Male Health.* London: Vermilion.

Carrol, S. (2003) *The Which? Guide to Men's Health.* London: Which? Books Consumers' Association.

Douglas, K. (2002) *My Stroke of Luck.* London: Little, Brown.

Fairclough, P.L. (2002) *Living with Brain Injury.* London: Jessica Kingsley Publishers.

Gray, H. (2003) *Gray's Anatomy.* Bath: Parragon.

Jacobson, E. (1964) *Anxiety and Tension Control.* Philadelphia, PA: Lippincott.

Lynas, J. (2002) *Cooking for a Healthy Heart* (in association with HEART UK). London: Hamlyn.

Millikan, C.H., McDowell, F. and Easton, J.D. (1987) *Stroke.* Philadelphia, PA: Lea and Febiger.

Ody, P. (2000) *Practical Chinese Medicine.* London: Godsfield Press.

Powell, T. (2001) *Head Injury: A Practical Guide.* Bicester: Speechmark Publishing.

Rudd, A., Irwin, P. and Penhale, P. (2000) *Stroke: At Your Fingertips.* London: Class Publishing.

Sieger, R. (2004) *Natural Born Winners.* London: Arrow Books.

Smith, T. (1991) *Coping with Strokes.* London: Sheldon Press.

Staley, C.I. (1999) *The Science of Martial Arts Training.* Burbank, CA: Multi-Media Books.

Tyldesley, B. and Grieve, J.I. (2002) *Muscles, Nerves and Movement in Human Occupation.* Oxford: Blackwell Publishing.

Index